Praise for Run to the Ligh

"*Run to the Light* shows us that running is the ultimate faith healer, restoring belief not only in oneself but life's possibilities. Taylor can't run but her spirit is with Laura every stride, every breath and every finish line."—Bart Yasso, member, Running USA Hall of Champions; former chief running officer, *Runner's World*

"There is death in the air, but Laura King Edwards defies it every step of the way, running to beat the odds on behalf of her sister and every child suffering at the hand of an incurable disease. Beautifully and thoughtfully written, this personal account of triumph in the face of tragedy will steal your heart."—Linda Vigen Phillips, author of *Crazy* (Junior Library Guild selection and New York Public Library Best Books for Teens 2014) and *Behind These Hands*

"Laura King Edwards's younger sister, Taylor, was diagnosed with Batten disease, a rare, degenerative brain disease with no known treatment or cure, just a few weeks before Taylor's eighth birthday and a month after Laura's wedding. You might be concerned that this memoir will be depressing. But you'd be wrong. Because of the author's dazzling use of language, because of her brave wisdom, because of her intense love for her sister, this book is powerfully uplifting. Prepare for an emotional impact: you'll discover, along with the author, how to find hope and meaning in the midst of life's ruthless complexities."— Judy Goldman, author of five books including the memoir *Losing My Sister*

"In this powerful memoir, *Run to the Light*, a talented new writer, Laura King Edwards, tells a vivid, realistic, and heart-wrenching tale of supreme courage, perseverance, and faith in the face of unthinkable darkness. You will be weeping tears of sadness at the beginning and tears of inspiration at the end of this remarkable, sweet tale of a sister's love and devotion. It is a tale full of beauty, power, and grace. Every page led to an inspiring ending, and I loved reading it!" — Susan C. Ketchin, author of *The Christ-Haunted Landscape: Faith and Doubt in Southern Fiction*

"Laura King Edwards's *Run to the Light* is an intensely moving, lyrical tribute to her sister Taylor, who has a form of a devastating inherited neurological condition called Batten disease. Laura was initially less-than-thrilled to become a big sister during her sophomore year of high school, and was at first resentful of her involvement in Taylor's care. Laura could hardly have known that those were the good days, when Taylor was bright, beautiful, and active. The disease made its presence known slowly, and Laura relates the intensifying feelings as the diagnostic odyssey led from visual loss to a much more all-encompassing disorder. The family even trekked from their homes in North Carolina for Taylor to undergo experimental stem cell treatment in Oregon. Taylor is still beautiful, but Batten disease has taken its toll. Today she can't eat, walk, or see. Yet she smells, smiles, hears, and loves. Taylor is still very much Taylor. In *Run to the Light*, Laura chronicles the family's battle against Batten, culminating in her efforts to run a half marathon blindfolded in Taylor's honor. It is a compelling and unforgettable story of the love of two sisters."—Ricki Lewis, geneticist and author of *The Forever Fix: Gene Therapy and the Boy Who Saved It*

"Laura takes us on a journey that is so compelling, so honest, so raw, so heartfelt, it's nearly impossible to put it down. Crafted with love and wrapped in vulnerability and strength, it's the kind of story that makes you want to stand up and take immediate action. I'm inspired and awed, and I know that Laura and her family are creating the kind of change that will impact thousands and thousands of 'Taylors' to come."—Jen Band, TEDx speaker and Playing for Others founder and executive director

"In *Run to the Light*, Laura King Edwards proves that one person really can make a difference in the world. Some tasks, from running a half marathon blindfolded to finding a cure for Batten disease, can feel impossible at first. But through hard work and never giving up, Laura shows that there is much to be hopeful about and anything is possible." —Jesica D'Avanza, runner, marathon coach, and author of runladylike.com

Run to the Light

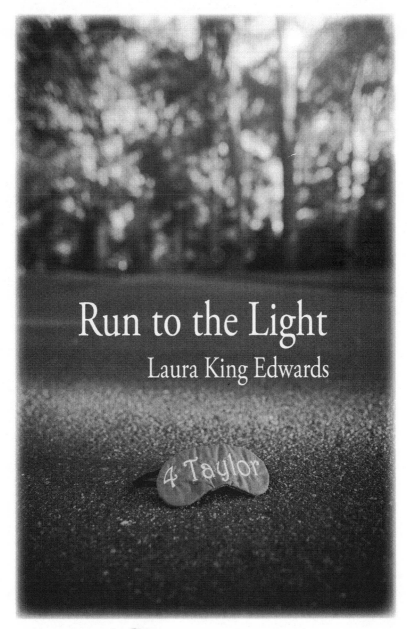

Run to the Light
Laura King Edwards

BInk *Bink Books*
Bedazzled Ink Publishing Company • Fairfield, California

paperback 978-1-945805-83-7

Cover Photo
by
Rusty Williams Photo

Cover Design
by

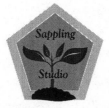

Bink Books
a division of
Bedazzled Ink Publishing, LLC
Fairfield, California
http://www.bedazzledink.com

For Taylor

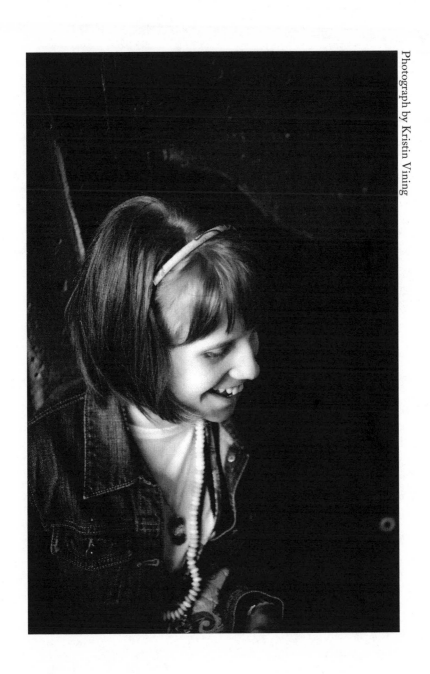

Prologue

THE POP OF the starter pistol shattered the damp air; it was time to go.

"I'm ready," I said.

"Run," Andrew said. My guide tugged on the bungee cord. I felt the coarse nylon and the cold metal hook in my hand.

The race had thousands of runners, but we were starting with the walkers thirty minutes early for safety. The bodies clustered around us talked about wicking fabric and post-race plans and their kids. However, we quickly left the others behind, and the cacophony of excited voices and rustling jackets and footfalls on pavement faded to a low din.

A chilly breeze carried the scents of hot chocolate and diesel fuel and sweat beading on brows. It was odd to feel the hairline cracks and the crunch of fallen leaves and the smoothness of painted traffic lines through my thick-soled shoes. I thought I heard someone shouting my name, but then the voice was gone and I couldn't be sure.

We ran down a hill. I felt the sudden grade change in my knees and the tips of my toes as they pounded the street, my legs cycling to keep up as the earth fell away beneath my feet.

The throaty rumble of an engine came up behind us and filled the quiet. "You have to slow down." The driver's guttural voice and the chatter of his police radio broke the calm. I quickly realized he must be the officer charged with pacing the early starters. Andrew was arguing with him, insisting we had permission to run ahead of the walkers, but I couldn't focus on the words.

I'd been training for this race for five months, but in a way I'd been preparing for it for years. Since my sister's diagnosis, running had sustained me as I fought my own demons. And now it'd become a powerful weapon in the war we were fighting for her life. I wasn't letting anyone—or anything—steal this moment.

Then the world was silent again except for the slap, slap of my laces against the tops of my shoes. Prickles of sweat clung to my back, and ringlets of hair curled at the nape of my neck. The curved metal hook of the bungee cord felt clammy in my hand.

Darkness had swallowed the light, but in my head I could see the finish line.

I filled my lungs with cold air, and I picked up speed.

Chapter 1

SOME PEOPLE SAY nothing good comes from phone calls in the dead of night, but I fear the worst from calls on a weekday when the morning sun still hangs low in the sky.

We found out my little sister was dying on a parched morning in the summer of 2006, just a few weeks shy of her eighth birthday and a month after my wedding. I sat at my desk at work, writing a press release, when my phone rang. On the other end of the line, my mother sobbed on my father's shoulder in a hot car in the parking lot of a doctor's office.

"It's Taylor," she said through choked gasps.

"What's wrong with Taylor?" A thousand sharp needles pricked my skin.

Taylor had something called neuronal ceroid lipofuscinosis, my mother said. I could hear her voice quivering.

Neuronal ceroid lipofuscinosis.

I typed the unfamiliar phrase into Google with trembling fingers and crumpled into my desk chair as I read the results. Words and phrases shot off the screen and straight into my vulnerable flesh like icy daggers, each one more awful than the last.

Rare. Inherited. Progressive. Seizures. Motor deterioration. Cognitive deterioration. Blindness. No treatment. No cure. Early death.

My sister had been dealing with some vision loss and struggles in math, but I'd never dreamed that these could be signs of a genetic disease—one with a scary name I had never heard and couldn't pronounce. My eyes blurred until I couldn't read the words on the computer screen any longer, so I put my head down on my desk, still clutching the phone to my ear. I waited for the nightmare to end and thought back to a happy memory.

A COUPLE OF years earlier, the summer before my sister started kindergarten, she'd helped me dig a huge hole in the sand during our family beach vacation. Using flimsy shovels and cheap plastic buckets from the Bargain Beachwear that sold ten t-shirts for ten dollars, we'd scooped sand out of the hole until it was big enough for both of us to climb down and sit cross-legged in the soft, wet muck at the bottom.

"Can we dig all the way to China?" Taylor asked.

"Maybe if we get a bigger shovel," I said.

She scrunched up her face for a second, and sunlight danced on her round cheeks as it shone down into our secret hideaway on the crowded beach. She set down the small shovel and took my pinky finger in her hand. "Can we stay down here forever?"

Then, I had smiled at the thought. Now, I felt that hole caving in around me, my mouth filling with sand, my lungs gasping for air.

That morning, the geneticist had sat across from my dazed parents and explained to them how an inherited defect in my sister's DNA, commonly called Batten disease, would begin its systematic destruction of a life filled with great promise. The doctor had said, "Go home and love her. Make happy memories. That's the best you can do."

For most of my life, I'd dealt with stress by running. And now, I felt a powerful urge to run.

So that's what I did. I said goodbye to my mother and placed the phone on its cradle, my hand shaking. I slung my purse over my shoulder and squinted through hot tears at our summer intern, who sat a few feet behind me and had witnessed the whole thing. I mustered a weak smile as if to say, "I'll be okay." But I had no idea if that was true. I stopped in front of my boss's door long enough to stammer, "I have to go." And then I ran. I ran in two-inch heels. I ran like my life depended on it, and maybe it did. I thought I might run forever, or the world might end at any moment. I couldn't breathe. I couldn't remember my name.

I couldn't think or see clearly, but my legs carried me to my car in the parking deck of the Charlotte hospital where I worked in marketing. I slid my key in the ignition and turned, then tried to remember how to drive. On the road, cars drifted past me in slow motion. Nothing seemed real. I kept my hands at ten and two on the wheel and tried not to fall apart at stoplights.

I WAS SIXTEEN when Taylor was born and hadn't wanted anything to do with a new baby. I had my own agenda, and it didn't include my mother getting pregnant.

My little sister arrived on a stifling August night the first week of eleventh grade. I was tying the laces on my cleats at soccer practice when Dad called to share the big news. "Now?" I whined after a brief pause when he told me their room number at the hospital. "I'm at practice, and we've got a tournament this weekend," I added quickly. "Give Mom a hug for me." I still haven't forgiven myself.

I saw Taylor for the first time two days later when they brought her home from the hospital. After school, my friend John raced up the stairs to the nursery while I stopped to dig in the pantry for a snack. He was peering over the side of the crib when I caught up with him a minute later. "Hey beautiful," he said. For John and Taylor, it was love at first sight. I was a tougher nut to crack.

Looking back, my sister *was* beautiful. God gave Taylor the softest, pinkest lips, hair like honey, and porcelain skin. Her eyes, a rich caramel color, were unlike any I'd ever seen, and they followed me wherever I went. But I didn't fall in love right away.

I stayed pretty wrapped up in my own life, though I'd give Taylor a bottle or change the occasional diaper when asked. I traveled with my soccer team almost every weekend, and during the week, I was more concerned with meeting my friends at coffee shops or going to concerts than hanging out with an infant.

But something happened to me the following summer. My younger brother Stephen left for a sailing camp on the North Carolina coast, but Mom and Dad convinced me to forgo a part-time job at the mall in exchange for watching Taylor for six dollars an hour so my mother, the director of education at a charter school, could go back to work. I balked at first; adolescent logic can be a funny thing, and folding jeans at The Gap sounded better than hanging out with my baby sister. But I relented when my parents said they couldn't afford to pay my soccer travel costs in the fall if Mom had to quit her job or put Taylor in an expensive daycare center.

Taylor and I shared lunches I prepared: mostly peanut butter sandwiches with the crust cut off, banana slices, and applesauce. We rolled a rubber ball down the stairs; we could do it one hundred times, but Taylor would burst out laughing every time the ball hit the entry hall's hardwood floor and went flying. We spent the hottest days curled up on the basement sofa, watching movies or reading fairy tales. She held my pinky finger when she slept in the crook of my arm. And without warning, one afternoon during the credits of a Disney movie, I fell in love.

A year later, I'd found myself in the twilight of another magical summer with Taylor. My mother had walked away from her job the previous fall after much soul-searching, and though my babysitting services were no longer needed, I spent every spare moment hanging out with my little sister for free. My friend John and I had become a couple, and sometimes he spent lunch breaks from his job at the neighborhood YMCA with us. When he came over we played video games in the cool basement after lunch. Taylor stood by our knees, slapping the coffee table with outstretched palms and giggling as princesses, armored turtles, and speedy hedgehogs ran across the screen. Some days I covered Mom's antique chestnut table with newspapers from the recycling bin, and we painted with finger paints till the bold colors coated the spaces under her tiny fingernails. By then she was almost two, and I got excited when she picked up new words. She couldn't say my whole name, but I didn't care. She called me "Rar-Rar;" I called her "T." I didn't want to leave her to go to Chapel Hill for college, but I did.

Taylor taught herself to read when she was three—she was super smart. I'll never forget the day she read an entire picture book to me in the back seat of the car while Dad ran inside Papa John's to pick up a pizza for dinner. Taylor's preschool teachers wrote the kids' names on their cubbies to help them learn to read, but my sister foiled their plans. She read all of her classmates' names aloud to them, showing them each where their cubbies were without them having to read themselves.

But Taylor's spunk was what I loved most about her.

In kindergarten, she got a learning game system called a Leapster, like the Nintendo Game Boys my brother Stephen and I had, but packed with colorful games based on things like phonics and spelling. More often than not, Taylor got the questions right. One Saturday night, John and I were playing cards at my parents' kitchen table. Taylor stood in the hallway, a few feet away. She held the game console in both hands, her thumbs beating out a response to a question. Her eyes were narrowed toward the tiny screen like angry lasers, and her lips were pursed. I don't think she had any clue we were watching her.

"Sorry, that's wrong," the Leapster's mechanical voice chided her in a singsong voice.

"Be quiet," Taylor retorted, like the Leapster wasn't a glorified video game but something she could smack the crap out of.

NOW THE PAINTED lines on the street blurred as I blinked back tears; I hadn't even realized I was crying again. I gripped the wheel and thought about another Saturday, when the air smelled like smoke and cider, and leaves scuttled across the driveway. That morning, Mom had called and asked if I could spare a couple of hours to work on arithmetic homework with my sister. My mother had been a piano performance major, and she'd never liked math. "You may have to be patient with her," she warned.

"I can handle it," I said, smiling. How hard could first grade homework possibly be?

"Okay," Mom said, not convinced. "Thanks for spending time with her."

In the afternoon, I took Taylor to a quiet Starbucks down the street from my parents' house. Inside, she ordered a decaf latte—she called it "milk and coffee"—with whipped cream and stood on her toes to survey the desserts in the glass case. Together, we bent over pencils and paper and ate snowflake cookies dusted in sugar, as rain pelted the pavement outside. But our four-dollar lattes grew cold while I tried every possible way to explain why two dimes and a nickel equal a quarter, and why five pennies equal a nickel. When I noticed the tears in Taylor's eyes, I put the homework away.

Though she read well ahead of her grade level, my sister never grasped simple math. The teachers and counselors had called it a "processing" problem. Now I wondered if we should have paid more attention to that sign.

THERE WERE PHYSICAL signs, too.

About the same time the following year, when Taylor was in the second grade, our whole family had gone to the state fair in Raleigh after the leaves turned the color of fire and the nights grew crisp. One vendor served hushpuppies in an old gristmill. As we walked outside licking honey butter from our fingers, we noticed Taylor fumbling with one outstretched foot to find the edge of the rickety stairs in the dim corridor leading out of the small building.

"Why did she stop?" John said.

"I don't think she can see the stairs," I whispered. I leaned in and put a hand on my sister's shoulder. While I steadied her, she located the stairs one at a time before emerging into late afternoon sunlight to stand safely in the grass. She'd chattered the whole time we were inside the gristmill, but now she was quiet. I saw my grandmother's face and knew she'd seen what happened, too. But none of us mentioned it that afternoon. Instead, we locked it away, as if by some unspoken agreement. Someone took Taylor's hand, and we blended into the masses streaming into the midway.

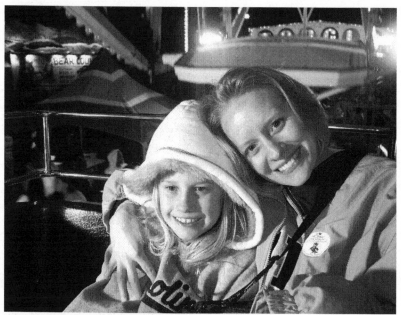

Taylor and Laura ride the Ferris wheel, 2005

We managed to forget about it then, but that awkward moment at the fair foreshadowed trouble with Taylor's eyesight. As that school year went on, I noticed something odd about Taylor. When I talked to her, she sometimes craned her neck sideways to focus on her peripheral field of vision. Later, I often caught her watching TV on Mom's ottoman inches from the screen, which ordinarily wouldn't have struck me as strange except for the fact that she'd be sitting at an angle, following the action out of the corner of her right eye.

That's what led Mom and Dad to take my sister to an eye doctor. Twelve days before I married John, that doctor diagnosed Taylor with retinitis pigmentosa, a degenerative eye disorder that can lead to blindness. We had separately convinced ourselves to face it later rather than let it ruin such a happy time.

Now, I wished the trouble with Taylor's eyes was "only" retinitis pigmentosa.

TWENTY MINUTES AFTER leaving my office, I pulled into my parents' driveway behind my new husband, who was stepping out of his car. In my emotional fog I hadn't told him, and then it hit me that he'd gotten a call from my parents, too.

"Where's Stephen?" I asked, noticing my brother's red truck was absent. It was July; he was leaving for college in a few weeks and had been working long hours as a groundskeeper all summer to save money.

John pulled me into his chest. His eyes were red-rimmed and swollen. "Your mom wasn't able to reach him. He might be on the tractor; he probably couldn't hear his phone."

Catching a glimpse of my sister's pink bicycle with streamers on the handles in the open garage, I broke down. I blinked through tears as John guided me inside and up the stairs. The house was quiet, and I remembered that Taylor was learning how to pirouette and plié at her ballerina day camp, oblivious to the tragic error on the single gene out of the thousands in her DNA. The plantation shutters were drawn closed in the master bedroom, where my parents sat shell-shocked on the floor.

"Why didn't you tell us?" I said as we sank down beside them.

My father was silent—his eyes didn't leave the carpet, like he couldn't bear to look at us. I noticed new lines in his face and more gray in his hair where dark brown used to be. My grandfather had died of heart failure almost four years earlier; Dad had inherited his insurance clients, bringing my family added financial stability we'd never known, but he also got saddled with the sole responsibility of looking after his mother and his mentally ill brother. And now—this.

It occurred to me then that he'd been more reserved than usual the past few weeks.

On the other hand, Mom's words tumbled into the charged space between us.

"The doctor called about a week before your wedding," Mom said. She kneaded the back of her neck, like she was trying to work out a crick. "She wanted us to take Taylor in for genetic testing. 'Just to be safe,' she said. The vision loss together with your sister's struggles in school made her suspicious. Another boy in her clinic had similar symptoms and had just been diagnosed with a rare disease. But I didn't want to upset you so close to the wedding.

"So we went in for the blood draw. Your sister hated the needle, but she was brave."

"Did you know what the doctor was looking for? Or why she suspected something worse?"

"I never even asked. I didn't think about that test again. And then they called us into the office this morning. They only told us it was urgent."

THE SUN SCALED the cloudless sky and baked the midsummer Carolina landscape. John drove us to a coffee shop close to my sister's camp.

As I stood in the cool, dim interior, I thought about that afternoon I spent with my sister at a Starbucks not so long ago. I tried to picture her peering at the baked goods, her slender fingers pressed against the glass case, or sipping her decaf latte through a plastic soda straw, a smear of powdered sugar on her cheek. But all I could see was tears welling up in her eyes as she struggled to puzzle out the answer to seven plus nine.

Mom wasn't ready to yield.

"Did you ever see *Lorenzo's Oil?*" she asked no one in particular as we sat down in a back corner. Her hazel eyes flashed, and in that moment, I saw more of my mother's true character than I'd seen in my lifetime. I'd spent a lot of time in the hospital as an infant, and my grandmother had told me stories about how Mom fought for me to get the best care. But we'd all been healthy for as long as I could remember, and I'd never seen this side of my mother.

My mother's third child was everything to her. Mom had Taylor in her early forties, when she'd already proved herself and saved the world several times over. She gave up all but a few volunteer posts when my sister arrived and quit her job scarcely more than a year later. I grew up on my father's grilled cheese sandwiches and kids' meals from the neighborhood fast food joint, but when my sister entered the picture, Mom started making a lot of home-cooked dinners. In typical teenage fashion, there were times when I resented my mother for waiting until the twilight of my childhood to slow down.

Now, I could tell that she was furious—she was ready to punch the lights out of Batten disease and anyone who dared to tell her Taylor's life wasn't worth fighting for. My heart swelled with pride. I hadn't seen *Lorenzo's Oil*, but I'd heard the story of the parents whose son had an incurable disease. They went to the ends of the earth to battle for his right to live.

"I'm not letting this disease call the shots," Mom added. "I'm going to fight." Left unspoken, floating wordlessly in the space between us, was the question: Are you coming with me?

MY SISTER'S BLONDE ponytail bounced on the nape of her neck as she skipped across the parking lot of her day camp and climbed into the back seat of our SUV, happy and unaware. She smiled and laughed and chattered about her morning and asked us to tune the radio to the Radio Disney station.

That's when we realized we didn't know what to do next. The afternoon and the rest of our lives stretched out before us like vast, dark unknowns. I tried to picture what I'd be doing had I not gotten that ill-fated phone call, but I found I couldn't even remember the day of the week.

"Where would you like to go, T?" I asked, hoping my sister could think more clearly than the rest of us.

"The Build-A-Bear Workshop!" Taylor's eyes lit up. "Can we go to the Build-A-Bear Workshop? Can we?"

"That sounds great," Mom said. John was already pulling the car out of the lot. As he did, I caught a glimpse of Taylor's face out of the corner of my eye. In that moment, she was beautiful—perfect. But she had just been sentenced to die.

At the "workshop," Taylor bounded from bear-making station to station. She insisted I build an identical bear so hers would have a twin, which is how we ended up with Cheerleader Bear and Cheerleader Bear 2.0. My sister never knew that I made a wish for her life on my bear's heart and stuffed it deep into the bear before sewing it up tightly—and it didn't feel silly at all. She never knew that I slept with the bear every night for months after the diagnosis, and she'll never know that the bear still makes me cry.

Chapter 2

THE FIRST TIME John had gone to the beach with my family, I noticed a long scar on the bottom of his right foot. He told me how he had cut it on an oyster shell when he was growing up on the coast in Florida. He still remembers feeling the white-hot pain, looking down, and seeing a massive amount of blood pooling in the sand, and later kicking the doctor in the face by accident. But he doesn't remember the moment before he stepped on the oyster, the car ride to the hospital, or his parents taking him home.

In that way, the days and weeks following the diagnosis were a shapeless blur. I remember specific details and intense moments, but everything else is fuzzy. My grandparents came from their home in Raleigh three hours away, but I don't remember how long they stayed. My Uncle David, a neurosurgeon in Greensboro and my mother's kid brother, drove two hours to see us in Charlotte the following day. I don't remember if we went out to eat, only that David held my mother while she stood on the stairs in my house and cried. One night, my brother's truck appeared in my driveway after dinner, and we sat at my kitchen table, his clothes still dusty from the day's work, and we talked about everything but Batten disease until our eyes grew heavy and he let himself out the back door. Dad made up excuses to meet me for lunch, like reviewing the investments I'd tweaked only weeks earlier or bringing me a clipping from the local newspaper, even though I had my own subscription.

Close family friends called and left baskets of food on my parents' doorstep. My own friends and coworkers from the hospital filled my email inbox with a tidal wave of messages offering their condolences. This was in the days before social media, but word travels quickly when a family gets slammed with a diagnosis like Taylor's, even in a city with over a million people. I tried to do ordinary things like exercise and go to work and make dinner. But my body felt as if it was not my own, and normal life stuff didn't make sense anymore. I found it impossible to care about decorating my new house or writing a marketing plan for a heart disease treatment when my little sister was dying of a brain disease.

TIME ALONE WITH Taylor had always been a treat. When she was two, we tagged along on a business conference with my dad to Toronto, and my sister and I went out for an adventure. At the bottom of the escalator at the hotel, an empty mall stood deserted before us like our own private, underground playground stretching into infinity. It was dark, but a soft yellow glow spilled through the security gates barring the closed shops. I stood at the top of the wheelchair ramp leading to the recessed mall and let go of the stroller handles. Standing behind my sister, I saw only the top of her fair head. But as she rolled away from me, she squealed and thrust her slender arms into the air. I ran to the bottom of the ramp, caught the stroller, and dragged it back to the top, only to let it roll to the bottom again. Taylor's over-the-moon shrieks bounced off distant walls.

I ran off the ramp and into the mall clutching the handles of my sister's stroller, darting in and out of the shadows and pools of light, popping wheelies on silver tiles and gliding across rows of gold tiles. Taylor's laughter rang throughout the darkness. Those few minutes of total abandonment were some of the happiest of my life. I couldn't have known then how much I needed to savor those times of pure joy with my sister.

IN THOSE HAZY weeks after the diagnosis, I held out hope that the lab had made a terrible mistake. It sounds desperate now, but I *felt* desperate. What if Taylor's results were borderline—abnormal but not bad enough to be Batten disease? What if we'd gotten someone else's results? I sometimes imagined that it was all one terrible dream. We were waiting on DNA test results from a special lab at Massachusetts General Hospital in Boston—at the time, the only lab that offered genetic testing for Batten disease. The results would provide genetic information about the mutation Taylor inherited from my parents—important, for example, if my brother and I or other relatives wanted to have carrier testing. I managed to convince myself that we might learn the whole thing was one big mistake.

Deep down, though, I knew it was real. For months, there had been signs of the secret hiding in Taylor's genes. At the time, they had just been too complex and too twisted for any of us to understand. I realized now that fighting a rare disease without a diagnosis was a little like trying to navigate a dark room without even realizing the lights had been turned out.

IT WAS RAINING the day the DNA test results arrived on a single sheet of Mass General letterhead. DNA doesn't lie, and I couldn't bear to look at the piece of paper that identified the two offending genes—one from each of our parents—out of the thousands of genes in my sister's genome sequence.

Batten disease is the common name for a group of rare, fatal brain diseases with no known cure. Kids like my sister can't make a lysosomal enzyme called PPT1. As I quickly learned, lysosomes are really important. They function like garbage disposals: in a basic sense, natural waste material goes to the lysosomes, where lysosomal enzymes break them down. But if an enzyme is missing, the waste material builds up over time. The cells get jammed with waste. The cells die. And when enough cells die, the person dies.

Most kids with Batten disease seem healthy when they're born, because there isn't any waste clogging their cells. Symptoms like learning disabilities, vision loss, speech problems, seizures, and mobility issues don't appear until later. There are four main types of Batten disease; the main distinguishing feature is age of onset, but my sister was a rarity among rarities. Taylor inherited the gene for the infantile form of Batten disease, which normally hits infants or toddlers. However, my sister produces a small amount of the lysosomal enzyme, which cleared some of the waste material from her cells and delayed her symptoms until the first grade.

TAYLOR'S VISION CONTINUED to deteriorate after that summer, although at a slow clip, and her struggles in school escalated. But for all the sleep we lost over her decline, if she shared our concerns, you wouldn't know it—and we told her as little as possible. "You're going to this doctor for your eyes," Mom and Dad would say to her, or,

e are some things happening to your body, but Ms. (insert name
erapist here) can help." We were never frank with Taylor about her
prognosis. Some families told their kids everything, but we didn't see
the need to burden my sister with her own mortality at the age of eight.

Instead, we watched Taylor tackle each new challenge without ever
asking, "Why me?" Even as her body started failing her, she sought
a normal life and never asked for extra help or attention. My sister
loved dancing and singing, Disney heartthrobs, trying on clothes, and
anything pink or purple. She liked to catch her Bichon Frise, Sunny, in
a bear hug and bury her face in the dog's soft, cottony white coat. The
disease working dark magic in her genes was all but invisible to most
people.

Not long after the diagnosis, an orientation and mobility specialist
from a non-profit agency for the blind began working with Taylor. Ian
was about my age and often wore shorts and leather thong sandals to his
appointments with Taylor. He had a relaxed nature, an infectious smile,
and kind eyes. My sister called him "Mr. Ian."

Doctors said it might be several years before Taylor lost all of her
vision. But my parents wanted to get a head start on the fight against
Batten disease. In addition to the orientation and mobility sessions
with Mr. Ian, they contacted a pediatric specialty clinic to ask about
occupational and physical therapy. They met with her neurologist and
pediatrician in Charlotte and found a Batten disease specialist in New
York.

One afternoon, Mr. Ian took Taylor to the mall so she could practice
walking with a cane. My sister went in style; she picked earrings that
matched her trendy top and carried a sparkly purse.

"What did you do with Mr. Ian yesterday, Taylor?" I asked when I
saw her the next day, expecting to get a rundown of what it felt like to
use a cane in the mall.

"We went shopping," she answered. "I bought Sunny a leash. It's
pink with paw prints. Want to see it?" She had soaked up her time on
the arm of a cute, older boy at the mall, using her own money to buy a
decaf latte—what else?—and treats for her dog.

She didn't say anything about cane training. In those early days,
Taylor hated cane training the most of all the things that went with
Batten disease, because it made her noticeably different from other kids.

She tolerated the cane lessons since an adult had told her she needed them (and she loved Mr. Ian), but otherwise, she avoided using her cane in public. She used her failing vision for as long as she could, and when the lights had all but faded, she memorized the layouts of familiar places, like my parents' house and her small private school.

Of all my sister's qualities, her resilience amazed me more than anything. When I was nine, Mom took me to the eye doctor after I complained that I couldn't see the math quizzes my teacher wrote on the board. I went home with thick glasses; I didn't fail any more quizzes, but I hated the Rec Specs I had to wear for my soccer games, and some of the boys at school teased me. I cried myself to sleep after the boy I secretly liked called me Four Eyes on the playground. But Taylor took her fading vision in stride.

It was harder for me to accept Taylor's failing eyesight and the more serious problems it foreshadowed. I didn't understand death then, and years later, I'm still not sure I do. John had to pull me away from my laptop the night the Batten Disease Support & Research Association added my sister to its online gallery of affected children. I scrolled through the pages of faces and names and hometowns and disease types and dates of birth and, for many, dates of death until my chest burned and my head pounded and my eyes felt heavy with hot tears.

The next night, I dragged myself off the living room sofa at a commercial break to rinse dinner dishes at the sink. John wandered into the kitchen for a drink and found me curled up on the cold tile, my back to the dishwasher, my shoulders shaking, the dishrag on the floor, forgotten.

I wasn't the only one who found it difficult most of the time and impossible some of the time to forge ahead into our new world with enthusiasm and grace. But Mom wasn't just devastated about Taylor's illness, she was angry. Not long after the diagnosis, Mom stood up and walked out of church smack in the middle of the minister's sermon. She didn't hate God or even blame Him for Taylor's illness, she told me afterward. She just didn't feel like praising Him that day.

The Batten Association support staff had given us contact information for other affected families. Many of these families offered helpful advice for our current situation and the horrors yet to come. But grateful as she was, my mother rejected the recommendation of some fellow Ba parents to tell Taylor everything—that she had a fatal disease and would never grow up. She refused to be labeled a Batten parent. "I never asked to join this club," she'd say. Instead, she vowed to fight for her daughter's life even as Google results and the city's best doctors and other affected families told her she was crazy to try.

I was in awe. In those early months, I couldn't match Mom stride for stride. Her grief fueled her fury; she wanted to punch Batten disease in the gut. I didn't know where she found the will to fight, but I never questioned her spirit. I understood enough about genetics to know how close I'd come to having Batten disease, and I knew I'd want her to wage a war for me, too.

On one of Mom's fighting days, she placed a bulk order for scores of hardcover copies of *The Cure*, a stunning account of how one man raised one hundred million dollars in an effort to save his children from another rare disorder. I was over for dinner the night the UPS deliveryman left a box the size of a microwave oven on my parents' front doorstep. We heard the whine of the delivery truck, the idling engine in front of the house, and a "thump" on the porch before the doorbell rang twice.

Dad peered at Mom over his grilled chicken and green salad. His eyes looked tired. "Are you expecting a package?"

"I ordered books for our steering committee," Mom said, as if we all knew what she was talking about.

I set down my fork. "What steering committee?"

Mom's eyes darted toward my sister, who was inspecting one of the fake gems on her bejeweled t-shirt. "You'll get an email later," she answered quickly.

The Cure, which inspired the movie *Extraordinary Measures*, tells the story of John Crowley's fight against a severe neuromuscular disorder called Pompe disease that affects his children, Megan and Patrick. At the time of their diagnosis, Pompe had no cure and no treatment. Like Batten disease, there wasn't a surgery or magic pill or alternative treatment that could stand up to all the horrible things that come with Pompe. But Crowley and his wife, Aileen, refused to accept their children's death

his job, invested his life savings in a biotech startup, worldwide manhunt for the scientist who could save ck's lives. After a long, hard-fought effort that included plenty of setbacks, Megan and Patrick received enzyme replacement therapy and bucked every dire prediction.

Several days after that box arrived on Mom's doorstep, she and her friends Martha and Stacy, like Mom both past presidents of community organizations such as the Junior League, assembled a group of handpicked women for lunch in Martha's living room. The faces around the room belonged to volunteer dynamos and business leaders, all close friends or contacts from Mom's life Before Batten Disease. Together, we made up the steering committee.

I listened and watched as my mother declared war on Batten disease and urged the rest of us to join her on the battlefield.

"The doctors said there's nothing we can do," she said. "But I'm not going down without a fight." Her voice cracked as she described our opponent, ticking off the symptoms that had crept into my sister's life and the awful ones yet to come. But her resolve never wavered. "Nothing about this will be easy. There's little being done for Batten disease. There aren't many kids like Taylor. But we have to start somewhere. Someone has to take a stand. And you know what? I believe."

The others sat transfixed, their homemade egg salad and pimento cheese sandwiches forgotten. I watched and listened to this iron-willed woman who'd given me life, and I knew I'd follow her to the ends of the earth to save my sister.

As Mom's last word—"believe"—hung in the air, a sudden breeze blew through the crimson and gold leaves that clung to the trees outside. I took a copy of *The Cure* for myself and gave one to each of the volunteers huddled in the room.

In that moment, Taylor's Tale was born.

Chapter 3

SOME DAYS, IT was hard to believe Taylor had a fatal disease. Her eyes were failing her, and on Halloween night, I worried she wouldn't be able to find her way up winding walks and front porch steps in the moonlight to collect her candy. But she skipped happily around my parents' neighborhood in her cheerleader costume, filling her plastic jack-o-lantern and not falling even once.

She was, in a lot of ways, the kid I'd always known.

When I'd married John in the mountains of North Carolina that summer, rain clouds had hung over our fertile corner of the world and kept our seventy-five guests inside following the ceremony. We crowded around the inn's small parlor, where Taylor and our cousin, Morgan, ruled the tiny, makeshift dance floor in their flower girl dresses. Taylor had insisted she be the "senior" flower girl because she was older, and even in John's arms, I couldn't help but watch my sister from across the room as she led our smaller cousin in a dance of her own creation, the world her stage. Her golden hair, twisted into a long braid, swung from side to side as she sashayed and twirled around the small space with her imaginary Prince Charming. I caught myself smiling when the girls got carried away and crashed into each other so violently that the jazz band lowered their instruments. The saxophone player had a pained look on his face, but he didn't know Taylor: clumsy and fearless. My sister inspected her silk taffeta dress; in that moment, the fabric's soft candlelight color caught flecks of light from lamps burning on the walls. When she didn't find any harm done, she popped up and kept going. Morgan scrambled up and after her.

I was so happy that day and Taylor was so stoic, it had been easy to forget that something was wrong with my senior flower girl.

WHILE MY SISTER defied expectations, our mother gave Taylor's local care team the Batten disease primer they didn't get in medical school and connected them with the infantile Batten disease specialist she'd selected to oversee everything. Dr. Krystyna Wisniewski was already in her late seventies, and her office was a plane ride away in Staten Island, New York. But she was the best. Mom peppered her with questions about alternative therapies and advancements in research during her visits to the clinic and the all-night searches she pulled on her laptop at home. She'd find obscure articles Dr. W., as we came to call her, and other experts had coauthored, and would email them to me when she could have been sleeping. "Might be valuable info," she'd say. "Please read." More often than not, it was.

Before the diagnosis, Mom and I had never gotten along that well. Lots of mothers and daughters butt heads, but we had epic battles. When I was a toddler, my parents and grandparents took me to a science center called Discovery Place. I wanted an over-priced trinket from the gift shop. When my mother carried me out of the shop without buying it, I scratched and clawed at her face and arms until blood ran down the front of her white sundress. We had to go home without seeing the rest of the exhibits, and Mom could never wear that dress again.

We shed less blood as I got older, but the fights were just as memorable. I took piano lessons for more than ten years. Mom insisted I practice six days a week for at least forty-five minutes and set the timer on the oven so I couldn't cheat. Not only did I have to play piano, I had to play the classics, while other kids got to play fun music from movie soundtracks and chart-topping albums. And while lots of students got away with just playing in the annual recital, I had to enter all of the competitions. The one time I didn't get a top score, Mom told me on the drive home that I didn't play to my potential. She was right, but I still fumed in the passenger seat.

But things changed when our little sister came along. Now, my heart swelled as I watched Mom wage a war for Taylor's life. I remembered all the times I told my mother I hated her, then climbed the rope ladder to my tree house or ran out into the rain or jammed the key into the ignition of my first car and sped off, leaving a cloud of dust and hurt in the driveway where she stood alone, her jaw set and her eyes hard. I hated myself for saying terrible things and wondered why it'd taken a fatal disease to bring us together.

WHILE MOM BECAME a self-taught expert on Batten disease, our steering committee began organizing the first fundraiser for Taylor's Tale. We called it Chapter One.

The plan was to serve cocktails and hors d'ouevres and give a couple of speeches in the caterer's home. I wrote copy for a brochure and reached out to Martin, the head of the creative agency that did most of the marketing material for the hospital where I worked. "I need your help," I said. Martin's "yes" popped into my inbox half an hour later, and he became the first in a long line of friends and acquaintances over the years who would support us in our quest. I was buoyed by the quick positive responses I would get to requests for help.

After the initial shock had worn off, our day-to-day routine was much the same as it had always been, except that Taylor had to learn to walk with a cane, flew to Staten Island for a checkup once in awhile, and had to take a lot of new medicines. One of the medications Dr. W. prescribed was a drug called Cystagon. The capsules were huge and expensive and available only by special order. They caused bad breath and leg pain and headaches, and they bleached my sister's golden hair. She hated taking them. But at the time, Cystagon was the best hope for her form of Batten disease. There was a chance it could slow progression, and that faint glimmer of hope was worth the side effects.

One night while I was over for dinner, my parents were having trouble getting Taylor to take her pills. Finally, Mom cast a pained look at my father, who shrugged helplessly, then sank into a chair at the kitchen table and ran his hands through his graying hair.

"You're sick, sweetheart." Mom sighed, her voice cracking. "You have to take your medicine." Though still beautiful, Mom had dark circles under her eyes and new lines in her cheeks. I couldn't help thinking how my mother, a superhero in the public eye, was at her most vulnerable in these simple, raw moments.

"I'm not sick," Taylor said, considering this. For good measure, she clapped her hand to her forehead. "I'm not hot."

Of course you're not, I thought to myself. Third graders think being sick means you have a fever and a runny nose and get to stay home from school. And Taylor wasn't sick in that way. But what could I possibly say to her at that moment? You have a degenerative brain disease? You have a lysosomal storage disorder, so you can't break down bad stuff in your cells, and the cells die, and that's why you're going blind? Mom and Dad gave you the gene for it, just like they gave you the genes for brown eyes and blonde hair? Stephen and I could have gotten it just as easily, but we didn't? How could an eight-year-old girl possibly comprehend her own mortality?

It was a question we'd never be able to answer. My sister was a smart kid, and she knew something was up; why else would she have to go to a special doctor in New York? But we fielded each new problem as it came. We didn't give Taylor a crystal ball.

TAYLOR COULDN'T SEE into the future, but we could. I saw it staring me down in the face the moment I Googled "neuronal ceroid lipofuscinosis" that awful morning in my office in July. That's why we scrambled to take her to Disney World as soon as possible, while she still had some vision.

The Tuesday after Thanksgiving, my grandparents came down from Raleigh to watch Taylor so Mom and Dad could drive to Orlando from Charlotte for the Lysosomal Disease Network World Symposium, which Mom had found during one of her many late-night Internet searches. It was an amazing coincidence that this symposium happened to be in the city housing The Happiest Place on Earth, as we could then combine the trips together. The symposium was a scientific meeting, and almost everyone there had a long string of letters after their name. My father must have known what he was getting himself into; a good sport, he went with Mom for moral support. I can still imagine his eyes glazing over in sessions. But my mother was a crusader and a sponge. She called every night with breathless updates.

"I tracked down a researcher from a lab at the University of Rochester in the bar," she said after day one. "I think he could be a good contact for us."

Early Friday morning, John and I drove to my parents' house with packed suitcases. Stephen was finishing up his first semester of college at North Carolina State and was in the middle of final exams, so he couldn't join us. But we loaded Taylor and my grandparents into my Explorer and pointed the car south for Orlando to fulfill my sister's dreams of seeing Cinderella's castle and meeting the Disney princesses.

Near the end of our six hundred-mile journey, my phone rang.

"Where are you?" Dad asked. "Did you know there's a space shuttle launch tonight?"

"Where are we?" I parroted to no one in particular. I was driving, but I'm notorious for my lack of directional skills, and in those days, I didn't have a GPS.

"I think we're about thirty minutes from the resort," John called from the third seat, where he was watching *Beauty and the Beast* with Taylor.

"We can be there in half an hour," I said to my father. "We'll see you in the parking lot."

When we pulled into the Port Orleans Resort a few minutes after eight-thirty, an orange glow tinged the night sky. My parents walked outside to meet us; Dad was in shorts and a t-shirt, but Mom still wore a suit jacket over tailored jeans and a conference nametag on a lanyard around her neck. We opened all of the Explorer's doors and stood on the floorboards just in time to get a glimpse of the space shuttle on the dark horizon. John lifted Taylor onto the Explorer's roof, where she sat cross-legged and grabbed ahold of the roof rack like it was the safety bar of a roller coaster car and she was about to go for a wild ride.

As the rocket began its ascent for the heavens, the dim glow grew to a bright, fiery orange. "Alright, T, it's over here, the rocket's lifting off now," someone called. Taylor laughed and clapped her hands. The rocket tore across the indigo sky, a ball of fire trailed by a streak of hot, white lightning. It grew fainter and fainter, and then, just as quickly as it'd ignited on the horizon, it was gone.

It's not every day that you get to see a space shuttle launch. For us, it felt like a once-in-a-lifetime experience. But it was obvious even then that Taylor couldn't quite see the rocket; she never looked right at the shuttle launch. The glow was too faint, too far away, and the night sky too dark. It was just one of many experiences Batten disease would rob from her.

THE NEXT MORNING, we had breakfast with the Disney princesses at Epcot Theme Park. Taylor collected the royals' autographs in a pink and purple autograph book and smiled starry smiles when the princesses hugged her or crouched down to whisper secrets in her ear.

After breakfast, we rushed to the Magic Kingdom. On a limited budget, we had just two full days to spend in the parks and a lot of ground to cover.

Because she had been diagnosed with a life-threatening medical condition, Taylor was eligible for support from the Make-A-Wish Foundation. If we'd called the team at Make-A-Wish that fall, we could have extended our stay. Maybe we could have dined with Cinderella in her castle instead of the cute Norwegian banquet hall in Epcot. Maybe we could have stayed at the swanky Grand Floridian instead of the practical Port Orleans. But while we weren't in denial about how sick Taylor really was, we wanted to have a normal trip to Disney World—to visit it like any other family.

So we packed a lifetime of memories into the two days we could afford, and we walked those enchanted sidewalks as anonymously as the thousands of other faces there to enjoy their wonders. We discovered the FastPass system for the more popular rides, so the lines weren't so bad. We couldn't afford the premium meal plan, but we ate our two meals a day like they were our last meals on Earth. We did Disney World like we weren't fighting Batten disease. We did it not under the pretense that my sister was dying, but that she just couldn't see well.

When we got to the Magic Kingdom that first day, Taylor asked if we could stop in one of the many gift shops. "I want a hat," she said. I figured my sister would pick out a sparkly princess hat, but instead, she selected a huge, plush chipmunk hat, because Chip and Dale are my favorite Disney characters, and wore it all day.

Taylor marveled at the park's giant Christmas tree, taller than my father's office building, with a thousand silvery ornaments. Together, we climbed to the top of Peter Pan's tree house. She clapped to the thump of the music at the daytime parades and squealed on the peaks and valleys of the Thunder Mountain roller coaster. She sat on Santa's lap and asked for reasonable gifts, like new Disney DVDs and a pink hula-hoop.

After lunch on our first day, we found a ride called Stitch's Great Escape on the park guide. Taylor had nearly worn out her *Lilo & Stitch* DVD, and the fifteen-minute "ride" was actually a show in a theater. It sounded like a perfect after-lunch activity. But Taylor disagreed.

"I'm not doing the Stitch ride," she said. "He spits on you."

"What?" Mom asked, with a hint of skepticism.

John laughed. "He doesn't spit on you, T."

"Yes he does. And it smells."

Taylor was an eight-year-old kid, and we figured kids make up stuff all the time. So we cleared our lunch table and walked to Stitch's Great Escape. Taylor didn't talk or laugh; instead, she stood with her arms crossed over her chest, her jaw set. When we got to the front of the line, an attendant ushered us inside to seats on the front row of a small theater. The lights were turned down, sound effects and voices started playing, and damn if Stitch didn't spit on us. Along with the other guests in the front row, we got squirted with water that smelled like curry as "Stitch" went on a mini-rampage in the theater. When we walked out into the sunshine fifteen minutes later, Mom turned to me and said, "T was right. I didn't like that, either." It wasn't until weeks later that I learned Taylor had gotten the scoop on half the rides in the Magic Kingdom from her friend Payton. Needless to say, I didn't question her theme park reviews again.

After the Stitch debacle, I couldn't wait to get Taylor to Space Mountain, my favorite ride in all of Disney World. I'd first ridden the roller coaster the summer I was four, when I thought the asteroids floating across the video screens in the long, snaking lines were giant chocolate chip cookies. I'd returned to the park my junior year of college and loved the ride just as much the second time around.

"Let's ride Space Mountain, Taylor," I said.

My sister shook her head. "I don't want to ride that one."

"Why not?"

Taylor pursed her lips, her eyes cast toward the pavement. We were standing in the middle of Main Street, surrounded by shops and restaurants and Disney characters. A horse-drawn trolley rolled by. The notes of a happy Christmas carol played in the distance.

"It's my favorite ride in the whole world. Will you ride it with me just once? Please?" I waited.

"Okay." Taylor's voice just barely rose above the commotion, but she never lifted her eyes from the street.

I took her hand and looked at John. "The cars seat three. You should come with us." To my parents and grandparents, I said, "We'll be back soon."

When we got to the front of the line, we sat Taylor between us in the car. Still euphoric over the chance to relive a childhood memory, I'd already forgotten my sister's hesitation. The car slid away from the launch area and into darkness.

On the first drop, Taylor let out a high-pitched, deafening scream, louder than anything I'd ever heard on a roller coaster; it filled the entire sphere of Space Mountain.

Inside the ride, the only light came from random, small pops of "starlight." I realized then that my sister, who'd become afraid of the dark as her vision faded over the past year, couldn't see the bursts of light John and I saw as our car zoomed around the track. As a toddler, Taylor was fearless. But when she first started losing her vision, she insisted on sleeping with the lights on. Eventually the lamp in her room wasn't enough to keep the specter of blindness away, and she began crawling in bed with our parents at bedtime. She'd known all along that my favorite ride would plunge her into black nothingness.

After that first drop, Taylor overcame her apprehension, and she laughed and squealed with the rest of us. But when it was over, she made it clear she'd had her fill of Space Mountain.

ON OUR SECOND and last night, we watched a parade on Main Street, near the foot of Cinderella's castle. "Look!" Taylor squealed, as one of the princess-themed floats passed so close she could have reached out and touched it. When fireworks painted the sky over the castle, she lifted her face toward the noise. I wondered how much she could see.

We stayed in the park long after the last parade float disappeared around the bend and the last firework sparkled and died over the gleaming turrets of the castle. We were about to walk toward the gate when Taylor tugged on John's sleeve.

"Can we ride the magic carpet again?" she said. Of all the rides in the park, The Magic Carpets of Aladdin had been her favorite. That afternoon, we'd ridden it seven times in a row.

We all looked at each other. Dad glanced at Taylor, then back at us. "Our tickets cost a fortune," he said, with a hint of a smile on his face. "They can keep the park open long enough for her to have one last ride."

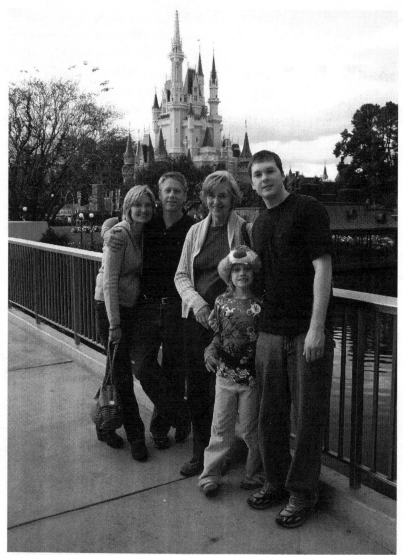

Taylor and her family share two magical days in Disney World, 2006

"Yay!" Taylor jumped a foot in the air. "Let's go!" My sister had no fear, and she took off in the direction of the ride, her long hair streaming behind her. I lunged out and grabbed her hand to guide her.

The ride was deserted except for the college-aged attendant picking at a loose thread on his Disney-issued shirt. "Do you want to ride?" he asked.

"She'd love to ride one last time," I said. Just as the attendant invited us to select our magic carpet, Aladdin and Jasmine appeared at the gate. Taylor stopped in her tracks and stared at the characters, spellbound. She'd seen them, or other actors in Aladdin and Jasmine costumes, plenty of times in the parks over the past two days. But this was different. They were here to ride *their* magic carpet ride, and we were the only other visitors in sight.

"Can we ride with you?" Jasmine said. She smiled at my sister, and she and Aladdin bent down to hug Taylor. Jasmine's huge gold earrings brushed my sister's shoulders.

The park that had been swarming with people an hour earlier was eerily quiet as Taylor tried to speak but realized she was tongue-tied. She nodded and took Aladdin's hand as he led her to one of the magic carpet cars. And for the next ten minutes, the attendant let us ride with the prince and princess, over and over again, as "A Whole New World" played in the background. When our dream ride ended, Aladdin gave my sister a kiss on the cheek.

The hard part hadn't started yet; I know that now. In the years to come, Taylor's world would go completely dark; she'd lose the ability to walk; even her beautiful voice would go quiet. Our trip to Disney World would have looked much different had we waited.

But for a few enchanted days, Taylor wasn't a kid with Batten disease. She was just my little sister.

ON A COLD, rainy Saturday morning in January, I took a bowl of cereal and a cup of coffee to our third bedroom-turned-office upstairs and turned on my laptop. I was still hunched over the screen in my pajamas when John knocked on the door three hours later.

"How's it going?"

I turned the screen of my computer to show him my masterpiece—an eight-page website with stock graphics, family photos, and a simple blog. All it needed was a story. "Not bad, huh?" I clicked through the pages of white space, hungry for copy. John kneaded my shoulders. "I love it," he said, like he meant it. "Just don't overdo it."

Another five hours passed. I wrote about disease causes and symptoms, disease types and rates of progression. I wrote about the history of research on Batten disease and the lack of treatments to save kids like my sister.

A football game was playing on the television downstairs when I made it to the blog. Alone in the office, I stared at yet another blank page on the screen, stretched out before me like a yawning void. What if I had the power to script the future, I thought? Batten disease felt so black and white. "This is what will happen," said all the experts and websites and encyclopedia-thick stack of papers the hospital's health librarian had pulled and printed for me when I told her about my sister's diagnosis. No ifs, ands, or buts. Plenty of people were ready to share their opinions on how we should react to my sister's early death sentence, but few had offered advice on how to fight for a real shot.

I thought for a minute. As another hard rain began to fall—freezing rain this time, so it sounded like a thousand tiny pebbles pouring down on the shingled roof above my head—I began typing my first-ever blog post.

Hello!

IN ELEMENTARY SCHOOL, I sat on a shaded hill overlooking the basketball court, devouring paperback books during our thirty-minute recess periods. My stomach stayed twisted in knots for days before my piano recitals. In high school, my soccer coach told me that my first touch on the ball would be a lot better if I could only relax on the field. Until college, I avoided talking in class—and when teachers forced me to speak up, my face turned a bright shade of red. I loved long, solitary runs and curling up for hours with a good book. I'm still the definition of an introvert—a strong "I" on the Myers-Briggs scale.

Taylor, a livewire, was on the opposite end of the spectrum. She'd always known exactly what she wanted and how to get it. She saw the whole world as hers for the taking and used just the right blend of sweetness and sass to get her way. Many times I could see her gears turning behind those sparkling eyes, devising a master plan. She was drawn to crowds and thrived on attention. In the center of chaos, there'd be my sister with a big grin on her face, her laughter filling the air. I had always admired that about Taylor.

Helping spearhead an effort to fight Batten disease forced me into the foreground, whether I liked it or not. Now, I wished I had some of my sister's unshakeable spunk. But online, I could hide behind my words. I'd always been comfortable sharing my stories, and publishing my work in what was then still a relatively new digital space didn't feel like such a huge leap.

Public speaking felt like more of a stretch than blogging, but as our first fundraiser, Chapter One, quickly approached, I surprised myself by imagining what I'd say to the crowd at the cocktail party, instead of how I'd get out of going. I took it all in—the stacks of freshly printed brochures, the wristbands from the Batten Disease Support & Research Association, the framed photos of Taylor for the welcome table, and the brief speech I'd written and crossed out and written again on a notepad, all scattered on my kitchen counter—and I got a rush thinking about the impact we could make. Lance Johnston, the director of the Batten Association, was flying to Charlotte from Ohio. More than one hundred fifty people had already replied that they were coming.

"Are you nervous?" John asked, minutes after we'd collapsed into bed and flicked off the lights the night before the event.

"Well," I said, stretching my arms and linking my fingers beneath my head. "No."

I thought about how, in the weeks after Taylor was diagnosed with Batten disease, I'd discovered I could walk up to perfect strangers and share her story. I'd learned I could be an extrovert when I needed to be. I'd seen that if I believed in something with every fiber in my body, I didn't have to be shy about it.

Chapter One was a blur of handshakes and smiles and hugs. I spent two hours talking to guests—many of whom I'd never met. I was totally out of my element, but when someone from the steering committee hushed the crowd and called my parents, Stephen, John, Lance, and me to the front of the room, I wasn't ready for the elbow rubbing to end. I wanted more.

Mom looked stunning in a charcoal suit. Her speech was upbeat and inspired. Lance had lost two children, one to Batten and one to a tragic car accident, and he wore the lines of a thousand miles on his face. But he was an almanac of information about Batten disease and offered a quick, helpful lesson on the monster we were fighting. I came next.

Right away I could tell I'd struck a nerve, but I don't remember what I said because of what happened afterward.

In the seven months since Taylor's diagnosis, my father had mostly stayed in the background, while Mom went after Batten like a pit bull. After I finished my speech, we thought we were done. But then Dad stepped forward and pulled a handmade Father's Day card from his jacket pocket.

"Taylor made this card for me in kindergarten, before she got sick," he said, his eyes misty. "I'd like to read it to you."

Taylor was always a girly girl, so it only made sense that she'd end a card to her daddy "Sweet Flower Dad." And after Dad read those words, the crowd stood silent. The steering committee member assigned to make the ask at the end of our talks finally appeared, and we melted into the back of the room.

Moments later, our Chapter One supporters donated $40,000 to the fight against Batten disease. I'll never forget the rush of adrenaline I got as the last guests departed and my friend, Callie, showed me the number on her calculator screen. I thought she'd miscounted.

That night, we delivered a blow to Batten disease. But Batten disease still took away time with my sister, at home fighting her own battle; Batten disease was still winning the war.

Chapter 4

SEASONS CHANGE, AND our lives change. The steely winter sky gave way to lush green leaves dotting tree branches and flowers carpeting beds of pine straw. The days got longer, the nights shorter. After the success of Chapter One, I felt reborn.

It was the spring of 2007. Taylor was doing well in her first year at The Fletcher School, a private school specializing in specific learning disabilities and attention deficit disorder. In addition to her regular classes at Fletcher, she was working with a teacher of the visually impaired—an expert on the educational needs of blind and visually impaired kids. Taylor and her vision teacher, Jill Fowler, were like two peas in a pod. They both had a dog and loved fashion and sparkly jewelry. The week after our fundraiser, Taylor and "Miss Jill" made me a pink and white heart-studded Valentine's Day card with Taylor's Perkins Brailler, a typewriter for the blind. At home, we baked cakes and decorated them with a thick layer of sprinkles; they were chaotic and colorful, like Jackson Pollock paintings. We threw birthday parties for Sunny and my dog, Daisy. On a family trip to the beach in April, Taylor ran through tidal pools and flopped belly-first into the sand and touched a stingray at the aquarium. Watching her unquenchable energy made Batten disease seem beatable.

In those days, it was easy to imagine that Taylor had retinitis pigmentosa and a learning disability, not Batten disease. But today was one thing; tomorrow was another. We never stopped thinking about how to get more good tomorrows.

The previous fall, around the time we took Taylor to Disney World, a California biotech company had kicked off a clinical trial to test its purified neural stem cells in six children with Batten disease at Oregon Health & Science University in Portland. The first part of the trial was a safety trial, a standard step in the process for a new treatment. The trial's first patient, a six-year-old boy from Southern California, was the first-ever recipient of transplanted fetal stem cells into the brain. In a safety trial, a treatment is tested in a small group of people for the first time to evaluate its safety, appropriate dosage, and possible side effects. While it isn't out of the question that patients in a safety trial will get better, helping them isn't the goal.

When I first heard about the Portland trial, I had mixed emotions. I knew they picked Batten disease for the safety trial because the sickest of the sick make good guinea pigs. I knew the trial's architects couldn't wait to develop and market their stem cells for more common illnesses, like Alzheimer's disease. I knew that if the trial saved the six kids with Batten disease, it'd be one heck of a fringe benefit—not the original objective.

But Portland represented a shot, which was better than nothing. After all, Batten had no approved treatments and a zero percent survival rate. Families like mine couldn't afford to be picky. I'll never forget what Lance Johnston, the Batten Association director, said during an NPR interview about the trial. "You can tell a parent it's just a safety trial," he said. "But that's not what they hear."

So Mom and Dad had put Taylor's name in the hat. The study team liked my sister's application enough to fly her and my parents to the West Coast and put them up in a hotel near the hospital. They sent Taylor through a series of long and complicated tests and procedures and scans with doctors and other specialists for the better part of a week that spring, to see if she would qualify. Taylor charmed the study team; the study coordinator looked forward to her singing, which filled the exam rooms and colorful hallways of OSHU's Doernbecher Children's Hospital, and the nurses knew my sister insisted on the pink—not blue—rubber tourniquets for her blood draws.

While Taylor got poked and prodded thousands of miles from home, I drained whole pots of coffee as I read article after article and listened to interview after interview on my laptop late into the night. The Portland trial became worldwide news when it was approved to move forward, and after the first patient, who couldn't speak or walk but could still see, survived the surgery, interest in the Portland experiment caught fire.

From reading about the trial and its first patient, Daniel Kerner, whose family was never shy about sharing their story, I knew that a surgical team drilled holes into each child's skull and passed a needle through the holes to inject the purified stem cells into multiple areas of the brain. I remember being surprised at how easily I absorbed the details of such a risky, grisly surgery with so many unknowns. On one hand, it was tough to think about putting Taylor, a little girl who looked mostly healthy, through such a terrible medical ordeal. But I already understood that even if she didn't *look* like she was dying, my sister *was* dying. That made taking a big risk a hell of a lot easier for us.

Not long after my parents and Taylor returned home from the West Coast, they got a phone call. My sister would be patient number four, with a July surgery date.

I don't recall what I said when my parents told me. I remember silently wondering how my sister would react to losing her hair. The doctors would have to shave her head to make the boreholes and inject the stem cells. How would we break the news that she'd have to give up her golden locks?

Then, a few weeks later, Mom and Dad got a second phone call from the study team.

"We lost our spot," Mom said when she called me that afternoon, her voice trembling.

"What?"

"Your sister got bumped."

"What?" I said again, because I didn't know what else to say.

"No Portland." She spoke in short, clipped phrases, and I knew she was trying to keep from crying.

I didn't have the emotional capacity to process what Mom was saying. The chance Portland offered may have scared the hell out of me, but it was the only chance in sight.

To this day, I think Taylor got bumped because she wasn't sick enough at the time; she was the only child skipping down the hospital hallways, and I think she was deemed to be too healthy for an experiment— too much of a risk for a safety trial. The study sponsor sent stacks of paperwork filled with fancy language explaining why families shouldn't have high hopes and more fancy language protecting the company if something went wrong, but it was easier and safer for them to select kids who *looked* like they were dying. These days, doctors and scientists are recognizing the value of early intervention; treatments are more effective, and more life quality can be saved, if we help patients earlier. But Taylor came along at a time when regulatory restrictions had a way of making it difficult to advance science and get treatments to the people who needed them most.

When Taylor lost her spot, I was devastated. It would be weeks before I realized that my sister's loss would be another child's gain. I knew nothing about the little boy from Pennsylvania who we later learned would get the fourth spot. He was already really sick—not so much of a risk for the study sponsor. But in those early days, I was so desperate to save Taylor's life, it didn't occur to me that other families were suffering, too.

NOT LONG AFTER the awfulness started, the Batten Association had given us contact information for another local family that had an affected child. That term always felt bland to me. "Affected" can mean anything. But it does not, as I quickly found on the day my sister was diagnosed, offer any leeway where Batten disease is concerned. There's more than one way to get to the end, but there's only one end.

Brandon Hawkins was a year older than Taylor; it was his diagnosis that had prompted my sister's pediatric neurologist to have her tested, too. There are more than ten forms of Batten disease, and unlike Taylor, who had infantile Batten disease, Brandon had the more common juvenile form. While the age of onset varies, the symptoms for each of the forms of Batten disease are similar. Brandon's father Chris had told us his oldest son was losing his vision and walked with a cane. Brandon's five-year-old brother, Jeremy, didn't have any vision loss, and by all accounts, he was full of energy. But he'd just tested positive for juvenile Batten disease, too. We still hadn't met the boys by the spring, but Chris had come alone to Chapter One and stood in the back of the room, his eyes shiny with tears.

In May, Chris and his wife Wendy organized a fundraiser for the Batten Association at the boys' school twenty miles to the north. Mom had stayed up half the previous night, making pound cakes for the bake sale.

It rained the day of the event. "Don't compare Taylor to the boys," I said to Mom as we speed-walked from our car to the school gym. I didn't want her to focus on the vision loss, speech problems, odd behaviors, or anything else that made my sister and the Hawkins brothers "Batten kids." But I knew in my heart that it was an impossible request.

"I won't," she said too quickly. She shifted the tower of pound cakes under her arm and put one hand on the door handle, hesitating. "Are you ready?"

We were late, and when we pushed open the heavy gym doors, we walked into a mass of people. But Brandon and Jeremy were impossible to miss. Brandon was tall and big-boned and had close-cropped dark hair, like his dad. Jeremy was a tiny, wiry ball of energy with a shock of platinum blond hair. Chris handed his older son the microphone as we slid the heavy pound cakes onto a folding table along the back wall.

"Alright people, listen up!" Brandon shouted. "My dad says we're gonna have a silent action soon!"

Chris smiled and leaned toward the microphone. "That's a silent *auction*," he said. "The items are on the tables along the back wall. Be sure to place your bids by noon. All proceeds go to the Batten Disease Support and Research Association."

"Yeah!" Brandon took the microphone in his hands again. "Fight Batten!"

While Brandon relished his role of sometimes-emcee, his brother Jeremy danced the cha cha slide, and Mom got into a conversation with Wendy. I drifted to the far wall of the gym, where a boy with smooth skin and dark glasses sat in a wheelchair.

"This is Adam," the woman said, his mother or maybe his caregiver, in the folding chair next to him.

With a jolt, I remembered seeing Adam's picture in the Batten Association website's gallery of affected children (that word again—"affected").

"I'm Laura," I said. "Taylor is my sister, but we didn't bring her today."

Adam reached for me.

"Can I hold his hand?" I asked.

"You can," the woman said.

"Okay." I took his hands in mine. They were hands that hadn't thrown a ball or built a sandcastle in a long time, but otherwise, the boy behind the dark glasses didn't look much different from the healthy kids at Taylor's school. Batten disease is a bitch, I thought. It steals everything—from eyes to legs—in slow, torturous fashion. Adam shouldn't be in this chair. He shouldn't be in *this* gym. He should be playing baseball or video games or riding his bike.

I lowered myself to the floor and sat with my back to the commotion. I thought about how, barring a miracle, Adam's present was T's future.

SUMMER. THE AIR smelled like grass clippings and charcoal and chlorine. On the weekends, Taylor and I spent long hours at the neighborhood pool.

We usually started in the shallow end, but we always ended up in the deep end, because Taylor loved the diving board, and going blind didn't faze her a bit. Though she hadn't completely lost her vision by then, my sister's world was dark enough that navigating a diving board could have been a scary proposition. But she came up with a routine: when she got to the front of the line, she'd listen for the sound of the person in front of her springing off the end of the board; then, she'd climb the short ladder and walk out on the board, her fingers curled tightly around the wet handrails. As she reached the end of the rails— about halfway out—I'd place one hand on her to guide her as she inched forward and came to a stop when her toes found empty space beyond the edge of the board. At that point, I'd drop my hand, and she'd launch into a cannonball, a pretzel (a Taylor original), or a nameless leap—her arms and legs outstretched in midair, her head thrown back in a laugh, and her eyes undoubtedly smiling behind the purple goggles she wore to keep water out of them. After resurfacing in the pool, Taylor always found the ladder on the side without any help. I remember watching this whole sequence a thousand times and thinking my sister had the best built-in GPS system I'd ever seen.

The diving board was a thrill, but it wasn't enough. Taylor desperately wanted to swim on the neighborhood swim team like the other kids, but because of her fading vision, she had to settle for swim lessons. She didn't cry or scream or ask, "Why me?" She just went to the shallow end of the pool three mornings a week and worked her butt off at the front crawl and back crawl and timing her breathing while her friends on the swim team swam laps in the practice lanes ten feet away.

In late June, Taylor's swim coach told her she'd made enough progress to swim backstroke in the team's last meet of the year. The night before the meet, Mom and Taylor went to the mall and bought the team swimsuit. Taylor was already wearing her new suit and swim cap when John and I got to my parents' house an hour before the meet began.

We were sitting on the pool deck when the sky opened up a minute before the gun for the first race. We wrapped Taylor in a thick beach towel and huddled in the snack bar while rain pounded the old metal roof.

"Listen, T, if they call this thing off, we'll come back and swim tomorrow," I said, rubbing her shoulders to keep her warm.

"It's not the same." Her eyes were cast downward behind her goggles, which she'd refused to take off.

She was right; it was a lame attempt on my part. I took a long swallow of my bottled water and pulled her close to me.

The rain never ended, and after an hour, the swim club sent everyone home. But a few weeks later, the swim teacher told my parents about a big exhibition meet and said Taylor could swim backstroke and freestyle. My sister shocked everyone—except maybe herself—by winning her heat in freestyle.

Chapter 5

IF THINGS HAD been different, Mom and Taylor would have been preparing for an extended stay on the West Coast for my sister's surgery that summer. Instead, in mid-July 2007, Mom and I packed for our first Batten Association conference in Rochester, New York. After the Chapter One fundraiser in February, generous donations from friends had continued pouring in, setting us up to award our first grant for research at the conference.

We took a cab from the Rochester airport to the host hotel and rolled our suitcases onto an escalator that climbed from the street level to a cavernous atrium. As we came eye level with the commotion inside the hotel, I felt Mom go limp like a rag doll. I threw one arm around her and grabbed the handles of our suitcases with my free hand. Then, I looked up and saw what Mom had seen.

Spread throughout the sitting areas, café, and main lobby were what seemed like hundreds of affected kids. They were all over the place. They were in regular wheelchairs and tilted, stroller-like wheelchairs. They had IV stands and tangles of cords and wires and empty, searching eyes. I'd read that Batten disease was a systematic shutdown of the body, but this was the first time I'd seen it in action. These kids couldn't see, but they also couldn't walk, talk, or swallow. Some of the kids—none of them babies—were in diapers.

Looking back now, I know probably fewer than one hundred kids were in that atrium. I know a lot of the kids were probably healthy siblings. I know some of the kids with Batten were probably, like Taylor, still "just blind." But all I could see was sickness and death.

We pulled ourselves together, eventually. We strapped on a hard shell fueled by Taylor's semi-stable condition, the confidence we'd gained from our early fundraising success, and a deep-rooted faith in the future that neither of us could explain. We talked of treatments and cures and building a better future for kids with Batten disease. "We're on a mission to save Taylor's life," we'd announce to skeptical parents and PhDs. We were so optimistic that some of the more battle-worn family members shook their heads, and one researcher even told us to temper our expectations. But we didn't back down. We skipped the family support sessions, instead grabbing the best seats at the research sessions, furiously taking notes and asking questions. That year's Batten Association conference was being held in conjunction with the NCL Congress, a scientific meeting that drew researchers from all over the world, so there were more scientists on hand than usual. We met experts from all over the United States as well as Great Britain, Germany, Finland, Norway, Poland, The Netherlands, and even Australia. After the sessions ended and most of the families went to the mall or the local minor league ballpark, we cornered the scientists in the hotel bar and asked more questions.

On the last night of the conference, we attended the Batten Association's annual banquet. Before we left our room to head downstairs, I slipped a check for $50,000 into my purse.

When we stepped off the elevator, we saw a long line of affected kids in wheelchairs and their siblings waiting to enter the banquet hall.

"What's going on?" I said, a little too loudly. I'd been laser-focused on making connections with the who's who in Batten disease research since we arrived in Rochester and hadn't paid much attention to the social events on the conference program.

"It's the parade of kids," the mother standing closest to me said. "It's the best part."

I stole a sideways glance at Mom, who didn't say anything. We made our way inside and found a table with a few researchers and a family from the Midwest. When the parade began a few minutes later, an emcee announced the affected kids' names. Mom's eyes were glassy and her jaw was set. I thought that if our table hadn't been so close to the front of the room, she would have left. It seemed as if no one felt the same way as my mother. Other parents scooted to the edge of their seats to get closer to the action. Dads kneeled on one knee and snapped pictures of their dying daughters and sons as healthy siblings pushed their wheelchairs down the aisle. I pulled out my cellphone and snapped a few fuzzy images of kids whose names and pasts I didn't know.

Later Mom told me she hated seeing those kids on display—that felt like it was more about the parents than the kids. "If they could a say, I don't think they'd want any part of it," she said. "There's nothing fun about Batten disease. I'm not putting my daughter on display like that." I thought that maybe the other families just wanted to celebrate their kids, but my mother saw it as a kind of pity. And true to her word, she never took Taylor to a family conference, even when the annual event came to Charlotte.

I was inspecting a dry slice of carrot cake with my fork when a board member stepped up to the podium.

"At this time, we'd like to begin awarding research grants for the coming year," she said. I looked at the program for the second time that night. The board member was a doctor from Kansas and had a child with juvenile Batten disease.

Mom and I sat quietly at our table until the board member announced our project. I couldn't help but notice that it was the only funded research for Taylor's type of Batten disease. Of the major forms, infantile Batten disease typically has the shortest lifespan, and many families quit fundraising—if they ever fundraise at all—after losing their own children. Without a lot of attention or backing for infantile Batten disease research, scientists hadn't made much progress in the past decade.

Dr. Sandra Hofmann's lab at the University of Texas Southwestern had discovered PPT1, an essential enzyme missing in kids like Taylor. But in the eleven years since, the research community hadn't had the means to do much with the discovery.

As I walked toward the podium to give Dr. Hofmann our check, I felt an unexpected rush, like I was on a roller coaster ride and we'd just made our first drop. With the money we'd raised in a few months, she'd have a whole year to explore ways to make the missing enzyme and get it into the brain. I thought about how Taylor was still running and dancing and singing at home in Charlotte. A year felt like plenty of time.

Dr. Hofmann, an MD/PhD with an oncology background, looked like a scientist. She wore glasses and conservative clothes and walked with a gait that ⟶ de me think she couldn't wait to get out of the spotlight.

⟋ for what you're doing," I said in a voice that only Dr.

the board member standing beside us at the podium

⟋ted to hug the person who had the best shot at saving

⟋t instead I settled for shaking the scientist's hand and

⟋ to her.

Dr. Hofmann's eyes seemed kind behind her thick glasses, but she didn't respond; instead, she smiled and gave me a quick nod, then turned and nearly ran back to her table.

The awkwardness of the moment slipped into my subconscious almost as soon as I stepped off the stage. I walked back to our table with my head held high, feeling proud of all we'd accomplished in such a short time and lucky that we had one of the top infantile Batten disease experts fighting for Taylor.

But the wind went out of my sails a few minutes later when we took home the Batten Association's first-place fundraising award, recognizing the top individual effort during the past year.

"First place goes to the Kings from Charlotte, North Carolina," said the board member from Kansas. "They raised $69,000 this year."

The crowd in the room—mostly families—gasped at our total. I was startled, too. I looked around at all of the admiring faces. Was $69,000 a lot of money? It'd scarcely been five months since that exhilarating moment when Callie and I added up the gifts from Chapter One—our first fundraiser. Had no one else raised more?

On the outside, I smiled because it felt like the right thing to do—and I *was* proud of all we'd accomplished, though I was grateful when the board member moved on to local chapter recognition and I didn't have to make a speech or go back to the podium to accept an award. But on the inside, I worried; if we could win the top fundraising award with a partial year's work, what did that mean for the future of all of those sick kids? What did it mean for my sister? As someone dimmed the lights for dancing and Mom and I took that as our cue to leave, I could think only about how far we still had to go.

After Mom was sleeping that night, I stared at the hotel room ceiling, my eyes wide open and suddenly blurry with tears. I kicked the heavy blankets to the end of the bed and ran my hands through my hair. For a brief moment, I considered switching on the small desk light in the corner of the dark room and organizing my notes from the conference sessions. Instead, I found my cellphone on the bedside table in the dark and deleted the few photos I'd managed to capture during the parade.

NOW THAT OUR first major fundraiser, our first conference, and our first major gift were behind us, we could have taken a step back to reflect. But when Mom and I returned to Charlotte, planning for two more events was already underway. Things were moving at a frenetic, breakneck pace. Some days I wondered if we should slow down, but then I imagined Batten disease catching up with us. All my life I'd been running; I wasn't about to lose this race.

While the steering committee planned a football-themed event with a heated tent and a band and an endorsement from the commissioner of the National Football League, a group of women in their mid-twenties—led by two of my coworkers—pulled together a committee of their own and began organizing a fairy tale ball for adults at a trendy venue in uptown Charlotte.

Fundraising events are hard work, and for the first time, I started spending more time trying to save my sister than being a sister to her. I'd go a week without seeing Taylor; I'd lie in bed and count the days and the months and the years the books said I had left with her if we didn't save her, and I'd dislike myself for all the time I spent sitting in volunteer meetings and working on my laptop.

One Saturday in August, Mom and Dad asked me to watch Taylor for a few hours while they ran errands. I drove the three miles to their house and plopped down on the sofa next to her, where she was listening to a Disney movie on her portable DVD player. I was watching my parents' car back down the driveway when I got an idea.

"Hey, T?" No answer. The opening credits had just started rolling, but Taylor was engrossed. I reached over and turned down the volume on the DVD player. "Let's get our nails done." Apparently, I'd said the magic words. My sister tossed the DVD player onto the sofa, slid onto the floor, and ran upstairs, all in one motion. "Where are you going?"

"I need my purse," she called back. "Coming!"

Fifteen minutes later, we were sitting in side-by-side massage chairs, soaking our feet. Taylor sat in the too-big chair, her eyes closed, a wide grin on her face. She giggled each time the roller bar crawled up her spine. She held still as a statue while the pedicurist painted her toenails with flamingo-pink nail polish.

I'd found a travel magazine mixed in with the usual trash available at most nail salons. "Hey, T," I said. "If you could go anywhere in the world, where would you go?"

"Hawaii," she answered with absolute certainty.

Instantly, a memory of Taylor and our cousin Morgan dancing in my grandparents' backyard, Hawaiian leis swinging from their necks, flooded through me. We'd gathered there with family and close friends for a shower three weeks before my wedding, marking the first day of the happiest time of my life. We ate burgers and grilled chicken served on the finest paper plates and dined on card tables set up on the lawn behind Grandma Kathryn's beloved back porch with the lazy fan and the porch swing that could put you to sleep on a stifling summer night or a frigid winter morning if you wrapped up in the afghan. The sun sank beneath the horizon about the time John and I opened the last gift and Papa Jerry polished off the last piece of cake. The leis had been Taylor's idea; she and Morgan hung them around their necks and chased fireflies across the grass, their bare shoulders bathed in the soft moonlight and their laughter in our ears.

Taylor was diagnosed with Batten disease less than two months later.

Now, my eyes watered in the middle of the nail salon as I thought about how my sister would never see the Hawaii she likely remembered from the *Lilo & Stitch* movies, even if we found a way to get her there. Right then, Hawaii didn't seem like enough for my sister. I wanted to take the whole world, wrap it up in pretty paper, put a bow on it, and give it to her. But she hadn't asked for that. In fact, she hadn't asked for anything at all.

IN THE LAST days of summer, John and our friend Callie convinced me to take an entire weekend off from my laptop and spend the extra time with my sister. Callie had been accepted to law school at Northwestern University, and she and her dog, Mason, were moving to a tiny apartment in Chicago's Streeterville neighborhood. "If you come to Chicago we can have sleepovers, though you might have to sleep with Mr. Mason," she told Taylor.

"Why don't we have a sleepover at my house before Callie leaves?" I said to Taylor, whose eyes lit up when she heard the word "sleepover."

That Saturday afternoon, Taylor appeared on my doorstep, carrying her pink backpack, Hello Kitty down pillow, and a case of DVD movies. She blinked in the bright sunshine, and I wanted to ask her how much she could still see, but I didn't.

John left for a friend's house when Callie arrived with Mr. Mason. "Let's make pizzas," Callie said to my sister, producing two bags of chilled pizza dough from her duffel and letting Taylor feel the squishy texture through the thin plastic.

My kitchen was a royal mess by the time we'd prepared three lopsided personal pizzas and homemade bubble gum ice cream, but I didn't feel like cleaning up as I watched Taylor play with Callie's dog and my dog Daisy on the floor of the living room, a dusting of flour on her temple where she'd brushed her long hair back from her face. After two princess movies, Callie and Mason climbed the stairs to our second floor guest room, and Taylor crawled into bed with me. She nuzzled close to me and curled her body the way she had when she was a baby. It was too hot to snuggle, even with the ceiling fan, but I didn't care. Having her next to me made me happier than anything in the world, and instead of sheep I counted all the hours I'd lost with her that year in exchange for long nights and weekend days on my laptop. I fell into such a deep sleep that I didn't hear John jangling his keys in the lock when he came home.

MY SISTER WAS not in the bed when I awoke to soft sunlight filtering through my blinds the next morning, but I heard plates and cups rattling in the kitchen sink. I shuffled into the kitchen to find Callie cracking eggs for French toast.

"Morning," she said, as if she'd been up for a while.

"Morning," I said. I rubbed my eyes. "Have you seen Taylor?"

"I think she must be upstairs," she answered.

"Oh, good—John said he'd sleep in the bonus room," I said. "So she's not alone." But something didn't feel right. "You know what? I'm going to go check on her."

I took the stairs two at a time, suddenly concerned though I wasn't sure why.

John was standing just inside the bonus room. His hair was mussed and he was wearing rumpled pajama pants, but he looked like he was in shock.

"What's wrong?" I asked.

"Hey, T," he said softly over his shoulder. "Come show Laura." Then he stepped aside, and I saw my sister had been hiding behind him. She had something in her hand.

"What is it, sweetie?" I asked, thinking she'd broken one of my shot glasses or seashells. But when my sister uncurled her fingers, she had what looked like two small, white chips of porcelain in her hand. It took several long seconds for me to realize she was holding her teeth.

"Ohmigod," I said, sucking in my breath. I forced myself to stay calm, because freaking out would not have helped me get Taylor to talk. "What happened? Taylor, honey, let me see your mouth. Can you smile for me?" She shook her head violently. "Please?"

"Show Laura, sweetie," John said. Taylor likely didn't notice, but I saw now that my husband was crying.

Finally my sister opened her mouth. The bottom halves of her two front teeth—both permanent—had broken off. "What happened?" I said to John, struggling to keep my composure.

"She must have tripped and hit the wall," he said, gesturing toward the half-wall that separated the main bonus room from the reading nook in the back. "You can see the teeth marks."

"Okay, listen," I said, turning toward my sister. "This can be fixed. The dentist can fix your teeth, okay? Can I have the pieces? We don't want to lose them." I watched Taylor's face closely as she held out her hand and let me take the lower halves of the adult teeth that had made her feel so grown up.

Later that day, Taylor's dentist glued her teeth back together. They never looked the same again, and in the years to come, the bottom halves would become discolored. But the cosmetic flaw never bothered me as much as the way the accident itself—something that happened because she couldn't see—made my sister feel. Even then, I knew I'd never forget how her face and entire body were wracked with shame.

WE'D NEVER THOUGHT the business part of fighting Batten disease would come easily either, but after early success, Taylor's Tale came crashing back to Earth that fall. We'd gone to Blowing Rock in the North Carolina mountains with my parents for Labor Day weekend.

In those days before smartphones, after breakfast each morning, Mom and I went to the inn's small business center to check email. On Sunday, we were about to head back to our rooms to get the day started when a long email from one of the fairy tale ball event planners popped into my inbox.

There'd been some disagreement over the appropriate ticket price for a gala with a full dinner menu and open bar; it was an expensive event, but some of the planners worried that their twenty-something friends wouldn't be able to afford to come and pushed to lower the ticket price, which our steering committee felt put the onus on the caterer to ensure the event raised—not lost—money for Taylor's Tale by covering a lot of the hard costs. It put me squarely in the middle.

The hurtful words in that email left Mom and me in tears. It started a months-long struggle as the gala planning continued. But Mom and I shouldered the emotional brunt to protect Taylor's Tale and my relationships at the office, since several of the event planners were also my coworkers. Meanwhile, the caterer shouldered much of the financial burden, enabling the event planners to lower the ticket price, which got more people to the event.

At the end of the day, it was a gorgeous evening that raised money for research, and a lot of new people learned about Batten disease. I have good memories of the ball, and all these years later, I don't have the capacity to be bitter. But the experience taught me a lot of tough lessons, including some I had to learn and relearn before I really understood. Anytime you face something like Batten disease, you eventually figure out who your real friends are. You learn that allies will come in and out of the picture, but you'll never get a day off, because this is your life. You learn that losing someone you love to a monster like Batten disease doesn't build character; it only reveals it.

AUTUMN CAME FAST and furious. By day, I went to my job at the hospital and worked hard to tell stories of our patients fighting difficult but mostly surmountable illnesses and injuries. I was inspired every time I heard about another advanced heart disease patient or childhood cancer survivor we'd saved. I never told anyone how much it hurt that my employer couldn't save my sister. By night, I dedicated myself to my blog and worked to get more media coverage for Taylor's Tale.

Meanwhile, I redoubled my efforts to keep up with Taylor's life in spite of Batten. Her school served students with specific learning disabilities and/or attention deficit disorder—both issues more prevalent in boys than girls. My sister never had more than six or seven girls in her grade, and they stuck together like Velcro. Fletcher's lower school counselor had talked to them about Taylor's disability. Years later, Taylor's best friend, Charlotte, told me the girls fought over who'd get to walk Taylor to her next class. They helped her navigate the hallways; she taught them dance moves and could recite entire movies. She knew Charlotte's favorite color was yellow. I used to worry that the kids would alienate my sister because she was different. But Taylor never acted like she was different than the other kids, and she never asked for special treatment. Instead of being alienated, she achieved semi-rock star status at the tiny school where the high school seniors walked the same halls as the fourth graders.

In November, the Taylor's Tale steering committee threw Touchdown for Taylor, our second big party for the fight against Batten disease. We invited everyone we knew to a mansion made of stone, which we'd decorated in Carolina Panthers blue, silver, and black. One of our committee members used her considerable connections to get the hometown team involved; they donated items for the silent auction and sent their mascot, who entertained guests when they arrived and breakdanced after the plated dinner. Another committee member was a friend of a friend of Commissioner Roger Goodell, who agreed to film a video for our event if I'd write a script; the video played on screens throughout the massive house, imploring guests to help us write a happy ending to Taylor's Tale. We raised $40,000 again and got on the local news.

We hadn't even had time to write thank you notes when my parents got a phone call from Portland. Mom told me Taylor answered the call and promptly went skipping down the hall with the phone, singing that it was for Mom.

The study team really wanted Taylor in the trial, said a faraway voice on the other end of the line. There was one spot left. Surgery would be in January. Would my parents take it?

WE TRIED TO pretend that Christmas was just like any other Christmas. Stephen was home from college, and John and I spent the night at Mom and Dad's. On Christmas Eve night, Taylor composed a note to Santa and his reindeer in an uneven hand. The note read like a grocery list, itemizing the gourmet snacks they'd find on the brick hearth, from chocolate milk and candy cane-shaped sugar cookies to baby carrots for the reindeer. Not long before midnight, she stood by the window in the family room and waited for Santa's sleigh to pass by in the night sky. Suddenly, she grabbed my arm.

"Look, Laura! I just saw Rudolph!" It didn't sound like a joke. I knew my sister couldn't see anything if you put it two inches in front of her nose, much less flying objects. But right then, what she "saw" meant more than anything I could see.

JANUARY 2008. ANOTHER winter. The sky was an ashen gray. Soon, my parents and Taylor would board a plane for Portland, Oregon. Dad would stay for several weeks at a time, but Mom would live in the hotel at the bottom of the hill for six weeks while Taylor recovered.

One night after work, I went with Mom and Taylor to our hairdresser, Debbie. Taylor sat perfectly still in the chair, but I knew she wasn't happy. She was so proud of her long locks; she almost never wore them pulled back, so they flew behind her like golden streamers when she played outdoors. Mom and I watched as Debbie braided Taylor's hair. When she was done, she made eye contact with both of us for a moment before taking her scissors and placing them at the top of the braid; and with one snip, my sister's long locks were gone. Taylor sat still as a stone, her face trained on the space beyond her own reflection in the mirror.

Debbie disappeared into a back room; a few minutes later, she returned, the golden braid in a Ziploc bag so we could donate it to a charity called Locks of Love. She placed the bag in Mom's hands and set to work trimming what remained of Taylor's hair into a cute bob. My mother had held it together since Taylor climbed into the chair, but she couldn't handle it anymore. She cried softly as a gentle rain began falling outside.

That was the last of our time together before Portland. A few days later, the trial sponsor sent a limo service to my parents' house for their morning flight. Not long afterward, John, Stephen, and I followed them across the country.

Chapter 6

I REMEMBER LYING on my back in the grass when I was a little girl and watching faraway airplanes draw white lines in the open sky, like chalk on a driveway. I imagined the planes were silver birds or spaceships; for a long time, I only saw them up close in pictures.

For my eighth birthday, my parents gave me a plane ticket for a weeklong trip to Raleigh, where Grandma Kathryn and Papa Jerry greeted me in the terminal. My first airplane ride was one of the most exciting moments of my life to that point. Two flight attendants gave me cookies and Sprite and a travel pillow for the twenty-five minute ride and promised Mom and Dad they'd keep a close eye on me. Three months later, I climbed aboard my second plane, this time bound for New York, when my Granddaddy Parks and Grandma Margaret took me on a four-day coming of age trip, the highlight of which was a visit to the famous toy store FAO Schwarz in Manhattan. I'll never forget the giant Lego soldiers towering above me in glass cases or the army of plush, motorized stuffed animals that roamed the tiled floors, bright balloons tied to their backs so customers wouldn't trip over them. Granddaddy Parks gave me two crisp twenty-dollar bills to buy Brownie, a husky I'd found while exploring a section of the vast store's second floor near the top of the escalator. Our housekeeper at the Hilton tucked Brownie in when she made up my rollaway cot in the mornings.

By the time Taylor turned eight years old, she'd already flown twice, but she was too young to remember family trips to San Francisco and Toronto when she was a toddler. Recent travels had all been for appointments with doctors in equally distant places.

Saturday, January 12, 2008, was go time. The winter sky turned the color of ink as my husband and I rolled our carry-on luggage down the jetway toward our waiting plane. We'd both taken a week of vacation, but our first visit to Oregon didn't make me feel like we were on holiday. Once we had squeezed into our seats in coach, I wrenched my phone from my jeans pocket and went over last-minute details with my brother, who'd started a new semester at N.C. State University earlier that week and was catching another plane to Portland from Raleigh the next morning.

Our airline confirmation clearly said we were traveling to Portland, Oregon, by way of Atlanta and returning home eight days later, with a connection in Phoenix. It listed our departure and arrival times and seat rows and numbers. But as the first plane pulled away from the runway and Charlotte's twinkling lights grew smaller in the blackness beneath us, I realized we had no true roadmap for the events that were about to unfold.

"This is a good thing," John said, sensing my anxiety as I opened and closed my backpack seventeen times even after the flight attendant had told us to stow everything beneath the seats in front of us. He reached across the armrest and placed a hand over mine, and I discovered for the first time that my hands were shaking. "Trust me. We'll get through this week, and T will be back in Charlotte raising hell again before you know it."

I thought about my sister chasing Sunny around the kitchen table, launching the contents of my bedroom down the stairs, singing into a plastic microphone on the brick hearth, and eating chicken fingers and macaroni and cheese with her pink polished fingers. I envisioned long lists of preoperative instructions and imagined the fingernail polish, like her hair, would have to go. My eyes filled with tears.

Before I knew it, we were touching down in Atlanta. After the plane came to a stop, we merged into the line of bodies emptying out of the plane. And then, suddenly, we were running, gleaming bars and fast food restaurants and shoe shine stands blurring, to make our connection.

I couldn't read or sleep on the long flight from Atlanta to Portland. Instead, I watched the little airplane-shaped icon representing our jet travel across the continent on the small screen in the seat back in front of me. It was mesmerizing to trace our path as we flew over Alabama and Arkansas and Colorado and Idaho. After those angst-ridden hours at the start of the trip, I welcomed the monotony. My heart rate slowed, and the tension in my neck and shoulders relaxed. I locked all of my fears away, thinking I'd deal with them on the West Coast. My mind was a barren wasteland.

Mom, Dad, and Taylor picked us up in a rented Jeep Commander SUV, and John and I piled into the back seat with Taylor. The air was

damp, and the cold fingers of the Pacific Northwest burrowed under my
jacket and chilled my skin even as heat blasted from the air vents.

My mother had always been good at holding it together when the
situation demanded bravery. The summer I was twelve and Stephen was
seven, Mom came down with a high fever, abdominal pains, and violent
chills; it was the sickest I'd ever seen her. Since we'd just returned from
a weekend of hiking in the mountains, Mom thought maybe she'd been
bitten by a tick and caught Rocky Mountain spotted fever. Dad was
out of town on business, and I rocked and cried in the corner of my
parents' darkened bedroom while we waited for my grandmother to
arrive and Mom shivered beneath multiple layers of blankets. We fought
like crazy in those days, but I didn't want her to die. Despite the scare
my mother stayed calm, managing to convince us she'd live even as her
teeth chattered and beads of sweat formed on her brow, and by the time
Grandma Margaret turned her spare key in the lock at the back door,
my tears had dried and Stephen was engrossed in a video game in the
rocking chair by Mom's bedroom window.

Mom didn't have Rocky Mountain spotted fever after all—just a
nasty virus—and her stoic strength hadn't changed in fourteen years.
T's surgery was less than three days away, but she had a composed yet
tough demeanor, like she was running a board meeting or speaking
at a Taylor's Tale event. She had a charged energy that filled the
emotional void left by my father, who seemed to be in a fog, as if
he'd drifted into some alternate reality to dodge facing the very real
situation at hand.

"How," I started, "have things been going?" I took off my fleece hat
and wrapped an arm around Taylor's shoulder. She snuggled into my
marshmallow jacket. "Your coat is poofy," she said, giggling.

Dad's hands tightened on the wheel, but he waited for Mom to
answer my question.

"They've kept us busy," Mom said. "Lots of tests. But we don't have
to go back to the hospital until Monday morning."

"The nurses always give me the pink bands," Taylor contributed.
I knew from talking to Mom the previous night that my sister was
referring to the rubber tourniquets the study team tied around her arm
for endless blood draws. "And I got a sticker today." She tugged off one
wool mitten to show me the rainbow sticker on her porcelain skin.

I squeezed my eyes shut and tried not to think about a needle or an IV tube breaking the surface of my sister's delicate hand.

LATER, AFTER TAYLOR was sleeping, Mom and Dad pulled us aside in the kitchenette of our hotel suite.

"There's something you should know," Mom said.

I looked up from my mug of instant coffee and waited.

"One of the kids died."

My stomach lurched. Goosebumps prickled my skin.

"She was number two in the trial, and she was a lot sicker than Taylor. They said it was Batten disease that killed her. It wasn't the cells."

Batten disease always kills, I thought to myself.

"So what now?" I said, my voice cracking.

"Nothing. We forge ahead." She took a deep breath and fingered the wristband on her left wrist, a small length of rubber that she wore as a daily reminder to "Be Joyful in All Things." Dad took a gulp of his coffee and looked at the floor. "They had to tell us," Mom added quickly. "But since the disease—not the surgery—was to blame, the trial goes on."

WHEN STEPHEN ARRIVED from the East Coast around lunchtime on Sunday, we drove toward the town of Hood River after picking him up from the airport rather than heading back into Portland. Taylor had a full battery of pre-op appointments scheduled for Monday, and while no one ever acknowledged it, we didn't want to be anywhere near the hospital on our last day of freedom. We didn't want to talk about anything related to the surgery, either—including the girl who had died. So instead we talked about my brother's new semester at N.C. State and whether his Wolfpack or my Tar Heels would make a better run in the latter half of the college basketball season.

The highways near our hometown are concrete jungles fringed with billboards and rest stops. But the road to Hood River wound through a national forest; instead of fast-food restaurants and gas stations, we saw towering cliffs dotted with old-growth trees to the south and the Columbia River and Washington State to the north. Thirty minutes outside of the city, Dad pulled into the parking lot at Multnomah Falls, a cascade of icy water more than six hundred feet tall. A footpath wound its way up the steep cliffs, but it was a cold, wet day, and we couldn't risk Taylor getting sick or hurt by climbing a strenuous trail so close to the surgery. So we settled for looking—all except for my sister, who couldn't see the falls but said they were loud. Later, after we reached Hood River, we floated in and out of warm antique shops and ate pastries. And we waited.

TUESDAY CAME AT once too suddenly and not quickly enough. An alarm clock rang somewhere in our dark hotel suite. I found my phone on the nightstand in the smaller of the two bedrooms and glanced at the screen: 4:30 a.m. For a moment, I thought I was dreaming. Then, I looked at the screen again and saw the date: January 15. We'd had this date circled on the calendar since that second phone call from the study sponsor. And now it was real.

We didn't have time for breakfast or even instant coffee. But I could barely pull on my socks over my cold feet; for what could have been minutes or only a few seconds I sat frozen on the edge of the bed in our room, lit by the glow of a single, small lamp, as my mind raced with thoughts about the trial.

In the eighteen months since the diagnosis, I'd become considerably adept at grasping the science of Batten disease despite my preference for humanities classes in college. In my head, I ran through the nuts and bolts of my sister's surgery. In a few hours, a pediatric neurosurgeon would inject nearly a billion purified fetal neural stem cells into my sister's brain via six holes drilled into her skull. Taylor would receive immunosuppression therapy to prevent her body from recognizing the new cells as a threat and attacking them. If the cells survived, the hope was that they'd engraft in her brain and begin producing the enzyme Batten disease had stolen from her, and that would, in theory, protect her remaining brain cells. The stem cells, if they worked, would be like a pause button. Taylor would never be the old Taylor again, but she might have a real chance at survival.

But to have a shot, she had to get to the hospital. And Taylor refused to do anything my parents asked her to do that morning. I remembered Dad, for once taking an active role, explaining the surgery to her as he tucked her in bed with her stuffed animals the previous night.

"When we go to the hospital tomorrow, we'll meet more doctors," Dad had said. "They'll give you something to help you go to sleep. When you wake up, your hair will be gone and your head and tummy might hurt. But your hair will grow back before you know it, and you'll feel better soon." The tenderness in my father's voice was a welcome foil for the nervous electricity in our hotel suite. But Taylor didn't respond, instead staring blindly at the ceiling in the dim room as she twirled a lock of hair around one slender finger. I knew she understood this was it; that surgery wasn't the same as a simple blood draw or even an MRI. I think my little sister, the bravest person I've ever known, was scared stiff.

And now, she sat stone still at the desk in the common area listening to a Disney movie on her portable DVD player, her knees tucked under her chin and her jaw set, while the rest of us scrambled to pull ourselves together. Each time Mom walked by the desk, she'd plead with my sister to get dressed. But by five-thirty, Taylor hadn't moved, and my parents' nerves were rattled. Getting a kid dressed seems like such a small thing, but Mom and Dad were ready to crumble. They'd signed their daughter up for an experimental surgery that was both super risky and her best chance on the planet, but it wasn't happening unless they got her out the door.

That's when John walked over to Taylor and put a hand on her shoulder. "Sweetie, can you get dressed?" He spoke so softly, I almost didn't hear him; but I watched with disbelief as my sister switched off the DVD player, slid out of the desk chair, and walked into my parents' bedroom, where Mom had laid out her gray fleece hoodie and warm-up pants. Three minutes later, Taylor was dressed and we were walking toward the hotel lobby where a hired Town Car, and the unknown, awaited us.

THE LOBBY OF Doernbecher Children's Hospital at Oregon Health and Science University was bright and happy, with lots of windows and colorful bird sculptures suspended from the ceiling. I worked to convince myself that this could only be so bad, that God had some great plan for Taylor, that this trial was bigger, even, than fixing Batten disease and that my sister was the key to moving the science forward for millions of people suffering from many diseases.

An orderly brought T a wheelchair when we arrived, even though my sister was perfectly capable of walking; John pushed her around the lobby, popping wheelies and taking corners, and she laughed hysterically. I pictured a long-ago night in an underground mall in Toronto with a clear-eyed, fearless toddler in a stroller; she laughed much like the blind girl in the wheelchair, and for a split second, I smiled. But then, I remembered where we were. We were in Oregon, not Canada, and as much as I'd prayed for my sister's acceptance into the trial with every fiber in my body, now that we were here—on the verge of taking what I'd always known deep down was a tremendous leap of faith—I was petrified.

I WASN'T THE only one who was scared.

"I don't know if I can do this," Mom said, shaking her head. We were in pre-op, just out of earshot of the bay where a team of nurses and nurse anesthetists was hooking my sister up to machines and checking her vitals. Mom was talking to Susan, a research associate at OHSU and the study coordinator.

"Yes you can," I said. "She can," I said to Susan, a little more firmly. Then, I turned back to my mother. "Remember what you said in the coffee shop? The day T was diagnosed?" Mom didn't answer, though it was plain from her face that she remembered. "You said you wouldn't let this disease call the shots," I said. "You promised you'd fight. This might not be the kind of fighting you bargained for, but right now it's the best shot we've got."

"We'll take good care of her," Susan added. Her eyes were kind behind her thick glasses, and her voice sounded like that of a good friend, not a hospital employee we barely knew.

Mom closed her eyes and rested her head against the wall. "I'm ready," she said.

Back at my sister's bedside, I watched her go to sleep. Her now short blonde hair, soon to be shaved clean, spread out on the thin pillow beneath her head. The tips of her eyelashes almost touched her cheeks.

Moments later, they took her away, and suddenly I wanted more time; I wanted to tell my sister I loved her; I wanted to hold her in my arms and I wanted her to look me in the eye and tell me she'd be okay, but I knew she couldn't do that. Instead, I fell in step beside my mother as we moved to the hospital's family waiting room for pediatric surgical patients, the rest of our family not far behind. I closed my eyes, and I said a silent prayer.

Is it possible to have complete trust in God? I wanted to trust God then. I'd often struggled with the concept of a world that includes Batten disease, and in my darkest moments, I'd questioned my faith. But I'd never lost it. You can't use words like "hope" and "believe"—words that permeated our vocabulary—if you've lost your faith. And right then, I understood more than ever that we had to have faith, because we were in a burning building, even if we couldn't yet see the flames. An experimental stem cell transplant didn't come with any promises, but it gave us a window. And if you're stuck in a burning building, you jump. Faith is about believing in a higher power, but it's also about believing that even a hard landing might be better than sticking around and doing nothing at all.

WE WERE SO drained, it was difficult to fathom that the actual surgery hadn't even begun. In the waiting room, Mom and Dad sank onto a padded bench in the corner. Stephen sat next to my father and stared into a space beyond the small bank of public computers on the far side of the room. My husband, who can't sit still when he's anxious, paced.

Oregon Health & Science University is built on top of Marquam Hill, also known as Pill Hill because it's home to three hospitals, on the edge of downtown Portland. While it's a pain in the neck to navigate, it has one hell of a view at the top. I gazed out a wall of windows, watching wispy clouds form over the mountains in the distance and trying not to look at the clock.

Not long after we arrived in the waiting area, we saw my sister one last time when a herd of scrubs strode down the adjoining hallway, rolling Taylor's stretcher. Lying on her back with her still-thick, golden hair framing her face, I thought she looked like a sleeping angel.

A hazy winter sun hung low in the winter sky when we saw Susan again. She approached us, kneeled down, and placed a sealed Ziploc bag containing Taylor's shorn hair in my mother's hands. If ever there was a time when I thought Mom might lose her composure, it was now. But instead, she just nodded a silent thank you and clutched the bag to her chest.

NORMALLY I'D DREAD the thought of spending five hours in a hospital waiting room, but I had no concept of time in Portland. Seconds and minutes, hours and days—they all felt the same. So when the lead surgeon, Dr. Selden, came out in his scrubs to report that they'd gotten more proficient with the injections and expected to finish early, and that Taylor was doing well, I was surprised that they'd made so much progress. And when Susan returned later to tell us we'd be able to see my sister shortly, I experienced a strange, out-of-body sensation, as if the morning had never happened at all. It was as if I was a powerless audience, watching someone else live my life.

They wouldn't let me into the recovery area, because I wasn't a parent. I went out of my mind sitting in the family waiting room with John and Stephen after Susan took Mom and Dad to visit Taylor following the surgery. It wasn't until they'd moved her to her patient room upstairs that they allowed us to see her.

If I'd ever doubted for a moment that my sister was sick, I was sure of it the first time I saw her after the surgery in Portland. She had dark circles beneath her eyes, her scalp shone beneath the harsh fluorescent lighting, and the six surgical sites where they'd injected the stem cells were angry and red. Her slender arms formed a makeshift halo over her head on the thin hospital pillow; her hands were wrapped in a thick layer of yellow and blue tape to keep her from pulling at her IV lines and monitor wires, and the tip of one finger glowed hot pink from the oxygen sensor.

With a clear lack of better options and a full understanding of Batten's outcome if we did nothing, Portland had become, in a lot of ways, our Promised Land. Reading about the trial for the past year and even seeing G-rated photos of some of the other kids post-surgery had almost made the whole thing seem like a fairy tale, partially because we believed in it and partially because we needed to believe in it. But the image of my sister lying in that hospital bed, fresh wounds glistening on her scalp, was real, and my mind suddenly raced with questions.

How quickly would the scars heal? What would her hair look like when it grew back? Would her friends still love and accept her when she returned to school in February? She would have to continue taking immunosuppression drugs to protect the donor stem cells she'd received even after she returned home. Would we be able to keep her from stomach bugs and the common cold—normal stuff that could make her really sick? And of course, the question that weighed on me most of all: would the surgery save her?

I stood in the doorway and watched as Taylor, still groggy from the anesthesia, regained consciousness. When she came to, the first thing she did was reach up and touch the back of her head. She gingerly felt different areas of her scalp, looking for hair and not finding any. She was still too groggy to speak, but the annoyed expression on her face said, *"Those sons of bitches; they really did it."*

From my spot in the shadows of the cramped hospital room, I cracked a smile for the first time that day. Taylor had just been through one hell of a surgery. But the sister I knew and loved was still in there.

MOM WAS SO exhausted we convinced her to spend the night at the hotel with us, especially after my father, who can sleep standing up in the middle of a crowd, said the makeshift bed in Taylor's hospital room looked like heaven to him and offered to stay behind. At the hotel, we went through the motions of normal things like brushing our teeth and washing our faces. John and Stephen flipped through the channels on the flat-screen television without ever really watching anything. Mom went to bed with a copy of *Traditional Home* magazine, but I suspected she didn't much care about the season's hottest decorating trends. I tried to write a blog post, but I couldn't form complete sentences and fell asleep with my laptop askew on the loveseat beside me.

Wednesday morning we didn't have a car service, so we piled into the Commander and made the climb up Pill Hill. Taylor seemed to be recovering well, but she looked like she'd head-butted an ice pick. Thick, dark blood seeped from incisions as long as my finger running along the top of her bald head. I thought about how squeamish I'd always been about blood and guts. I passed out when an emergency medical technician sat on the edge of my seventh grade health teacher's desk and shared stories about what he did in the back of his ambulance, and to this day John warns me to look away during gory movie scenes. But Taylor's wounds didn't bother me in that way at all.

By the time John, Stephen, and I returned from the hospital lobby with steaming lattes, my father was engrossed in a newspaper he'd brought from Charlotte, which meant it was at least a week old. Mom was already camped out in the standard-issue, vinyl-upholstered rocking chair next to my sleeping sister's bed; she alternated between answering emails on her laptop and knitting a scarf, something she'd picked up to pass the time in Portland.

"Dr. Steiner dropped by," Mom said.

Dr. Steiner, a pediatrician specializing in genetics and one of the study's principal investigators, had a soft voice that was perfect for scared kids in the hospital. Mom and Dad had told me Dr. Steiner and coordinator Susan were the closest things we had to a friend in Portland.

"What did he say?" I said in a voice that dripped with guilt for missing the doctor, even though the coffee run had been Dad's idea.

"Everything looks good right now," Mom said, a tired smile tugging at her face and crinkling the corners of her eyes. She didn't look at me when she answered, instead twisting in her chair to gaze at Taylor and placing a hand on the blankets that covered the cords and wires tracking her every move for the unit nurses and study team. She shook her head. "It's a wonder the surgery happened. Susan told me last night they were on the phone with the FDA in the OR, waiting for the all-clear."

"Because the other girl died?"

Heavy silence.

"Because the other girl died." Something changed in my mother's face then, and I knew we were done talking about the trial for a while. "But that part's over now. There isn't anything exciting happening this morning, and your sister will probably sleep most of the day. Why don't you three go out and do something fun?"

"We should stay," I said in an uncertain tone, but Mom was shaking her head.

"Don't take this the wrong way, but there's nothing you can do to help her or Dad and me right now," she said. "Get some fresh air for a couple of hours. We'll need you later."

Winter coats rustled and car keys jingled somewhere behind me as John and Stephen stood to leave. But I didn't move.

"Don't worry," Mom said more firmly, not taking her eyes off Taylor. "When you get back, I'll have a full report to share and Miss T will be ready to antagonize your brother."

FOR THE TIME being, I convinced myself my sister would be okay. I told myself the scary part was over—that Taylor just needed to rest and before we knew it she'd be sporting a full head of hair and singing Hannah Montana songs at the top of her lungs. We fired up the heat in the Commander in a far corner of the hospital parking deck and pulled out one of the Oregon travel books Dad had bought at Powell's City of Books, a Portland landmark and the world's largest bookstore. After a brief debate, we decided on Cannon Beach, a small coastal town and home of the iconic Haystack Rock whose seashore provided the dramatic scenery in the movie *The Goonies*.

The passage to Cannon Beach from Portland travels over the Cascade Range. Douglas firs lined the road on either side, and fresh snow powdered every needle. In a clearing, I took a picture of distant Mount Jefferson, and John and Stephen threw snowballs. It wasn't until much later that I was struck by how easily we slipped into our old selves in moments like this even as my sister lay in a hospital bed. I hadn't realized how much I needed a mental break from the intense emotions of the week.

When we arrived in Cannon Beach, we shed our winter coats and shared a pizza in a restaurant overlooking the Pacific Ocean. Our shadows were lengthening when we stepped onto the sand. In my favorite picture from that trip, John and Stephen are walking toward the great Haystack Rock soaring more than two hundred feet into the sky; their silhouettes, like the rock, are jet-black against a landscape so bright it could be heaven, or the end of the world.

It was a good day.

"SHE'S A CHATTERBOX," said the redheaded nurse leaving Taylor's room when we arrived back at the hospital that night.

"She is?" I said, thinking T hadn't so much as moved an eyelid before we left that morning.

"Oh yes," she replied. "She's had all of us laughing."

"That's just like her," I said after a few seconds. "I can't wait to see her." I said goodnight to the nurse and walked into the room with my hands jammed in the pockets of my coat, still stiff with cold. John and Stephen followed close behind.

Stuffed animals and paperback books and handmade cards from the hospital's child life staff and friends at home decorated the windowsill. Oblivious to the relative commotion, Dad napped on the daybed in a contorted position, his pullover fleece hiked up to cover half his face from the glaring hospital room lights. Mom looked like she hadn't moved from the rocking chair next to my sister's bed since the morning, though she'd put the computer away. Her bag of yarn and knitting needles sat open on the floor nearby, and a new scarf fell across her lap in soft waves of cobalt, fuchsia, and plum.

"'You might have seen a housefly, maybe even a superfly, but I bet you ain't never seen a donkeyfly.'" It took me a moment to realize Taylor was quoting the movie *Shrek*; I twisted to look at the television, where Donkey was explaining the finer points of donkey science to Shrek the big green ogre.

My sister was on her back, the blood pressure and oxygen monitors and PICC line and IV machines around her humming softly beneath the din of the movie playing on the television near the ceiling. She still had dark circles under her eyes and electrodes all over her body, and she seemed thinner beneath the light green hospital gown. The wounds on her head almost seemed worse, as if they'd had time to ripen under the hospital room's unforgiving lights. They looked like something out of a horror movie—scary for a nine-year-old kid. For a split second, I was thankful my sister was now blind, because she couldn't see what Batten disease had done to her.

"I ain't *never* seen a donkeyfly," I agreed. I plopped down on the end of the hospital bed and found my sister's socked feet beneath the blankets. "What's up, T?"

"Shrek's an ogre. He smells and he burps a lot."

"He sure does. What about the princess?"

"She's pretty. But she's afraid of the dark. I don't like the dark."

"It's okay to be afraid of the dark," I said, stretching out on the thin mattress beside my little sister. "I don't like the dark, either." And as

Donkey and the smelly, burping ogre and his princess set off on their great journey, I drifted into a dreamless sleep.

SHE HAD SOME of her spunk back, but Taylor still looked terrible on Thursday morning. No one in my family had ever had cancer, but I thought maybe she looked like a chemo patient who'd put her head through a windshield. I couldn't stop thinking about how my sister looked before Portland. She didn't *look* sick. She was blind, but even that wasn't always immediately obvious because she was so good at accommodating for her visual handicap. She still ran and jumped and danced and sang and did most of the things normal kids do. She had a gorgeous complexion and didn't catch common illnesses any more than the next kid. Still, she was dying. Batten disease was a sneaky bastard, I'd decided.

My sister's eyes fluttered open when coordinator Susan stopped by after breakfast.

"How's everyone doing?" Susan said. Her gray hair was tousled and her glasses a little lopsided, and the pockets of her lab coat were stuffed with spiral notebooks and crumpled papers and pens. She had a sense of ordered chaos about her, but I liked that.

"I think Miss T will be ready to get out of here tomorrow," Mom answered, leaning over the bed and smiling at Taylor, who was rubbing one eye.

Susan nodded. "That's the plan. Dr. Steiner and Dr. Koch will be by this afternoon to see her and talk with you and Jim."

"You're breaking out of this place, T," Stephen sang. "And when you do, we be makin' waffles!" Taylor still looked like she was half-asleep, but she giggled at the *Shrek* reference.

WHEN SUSAN LEFT, Mom and Dad insisted the three of us leave, too. "Look," Mom said. "We survived yesterday. We'll survive today. And it's really better not to have a crowd in here when the doctors stop by. I'll fill you in later." So after buying steaming lattes and pastries for my parents and watching half of *Cinderella* with Taylor, we reluctantly went back out into the cold and pointed the Commander for Mount Hood, the highest mountain in Oregon.

Mount Hood, huge and silent on the horizon, watches over the city like a snowy sentry. It's only fifty miles from Portland, but it took us several hours to navigate the frozen forest of the Cascade Range. I couldn't help but notice that nobody uttered Taylor's name as our SUV wound through the towering evergreens covered with fresh snow. We talked about meaningless things mostly, like the football playoffs and video games.

By the time we reached the Timberline Lodge at the end of Mount Hood's frozen road, I was restless. I felt a sudden urge to run, my go-to de-stressor, but I was wearing heavy boots and the snow came to my waist. Instead, I sipped on a ten-dollar hot chocolate with real whipped cream and chocolate shavings and cinnamon sticks for straws and watched skiers cascade down the mountain's sheer slopes. Thousands of feet above us, they looked like tiny black stick figures against the sparkling white snow. In my imagination, we were there on family vacation, and Taylor was on the bunny slopes with my father. Behind the mountain, the sky was an impossible shade of blue.

Inside the lodge, I watched families with children eating lunch in the café and playing checkers by the fire and comparing notes on their morning ski runs. In a bizarre daydream, I thought I saw my sister, but before we cut off her long hair for the surgery. She was wearing a hot pink ski bib and a matching pink scarf and mittens and fuzzy earmuffs. She was listening to music and eating a ginger molasses cookie, like the ones we often baked for Christmas. But when she turned around to face us, I realized that girl didn't look like Taylor at all, and I remembered my sister was lying in a hospital bed fifty miles away in Portland, and she didn't have any of her hair and wouldn't be cleared to ski in a million years.

WE DROVE STRAIGHT to OHSU when we returned to Portland that night. Taylor was sitting upright in her bed for the first time since the surgery.

"What's up, T?" I dropped my bag in a chair and slung an arm around her shoulder.

"Hey Laura," she said cheerfully, like she hadn't been stuck in a ten-by-ten box for three days. "Look at all the cool stuff I got." It seemed she'd gotten all kinds of craft supplies and other goodies in care packages from friends and family back home. I felt a surge of love for the angels who'd thought to send these items in advance so my sister would get mail at the hospital before she was discharged.

Taylor waited for me to survey the cards and multicolored pipe cleaners and construction paper scattered across her plastic tray table. I pulled up a chair and took off my gloves. Together, we built a snowman from pink Play-Doh and set it on the windowsill so it could see the world.

THE NEXT MORNING when we arrived at the hospital, Taylor looked ready to run laps around her tiny room. She wore a pink and purple fleece hat, a gift from the family of Daniel Kerner, the first trial patient. It reminded me of the hats medieval court jesters wore. A rerun of *Hannah Montana* played on the television.

"Good morning," Mom said from the rocking chair. After two nights at our hotel, she'd taken night shift, insisting Dad get a break from sleeping like a sardine on the hospital room's stiff bed. My mother often manages to look better than she feels, but I wondered how much she'd slept.

Taylor grinned when Mom greeted us. "The doctor said I get to leave today."

I looked at my mother for confirmation; she nodded. "We should be released this afternoon. I told Taylor we could go somewhere special for dinner to celebrate."

My sister raised her head from her tray table, where she was stringing plastic beads onto a wire necklace. "We're going out for pizza. I'm making a necklace. Laura—do you want one?"

"Sure." I walked to the window; the sky that had been so blue when we sipped hot chocolates on Mount Hood was the color of ash.

I stood with my back to my sister, counting the needles on the towering evergreens that surround OHSU, searching for the place where the world ended and heaven began, trying to picture where we'd go from here.

My sister made a pipe cleaner spider with my brother while one of the nurses went over discharge instructions with my parents. Most of them were things we'd already heard from Susan and the doctors, like the specifics of the potent immunosuppression drug they'd prescribed to protect the donor cells and all of the things my sister wouldn't be able to do for the next year while she took the drug, like swim in the lake.

She had a little energy by this time, but my sister and John weren't popping wheelies in the wheelchair when we passed through the lobby of Doernbecher Children's Hospital to leave. Bundled into a cheetah-print coat and wearing a pink scarf, boots, and a hat that hid her scars, Taylor looked triumphant yet tragically ill. She'd obviously lost weight during her three-plus days in the hospital, and her eyes were still sunken and ringed by dark circles. I thought about how she'd always hated pulling her hair back; I missed the sight of her golden locks framing her face. But in a moment of clarity, I discovered that in spite of everything, my sister had an enormous grin on her face. A smile played on my lips as I tried not to cry.

"I love you, T," I said simply, softly. "Let's get out of here."

And that's what we did.

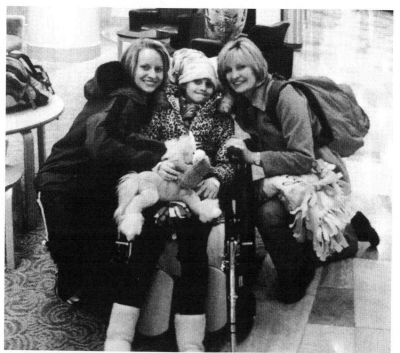

Taylor's triumphant discharge following brain surgery in Portland, 2008

Chapter 7

TAYLOR SPENT A month recovering in the tiny apartment at the foot of Pill Hill. Under the watchful eyes of my parents and her doctors and nurses at the hospital on the hill, she regained some of her strength and adjusted to the powerful drugs protecting the stem cells that had been injected into her brain.

When my sister finally came home from Portland on a cold night in February, she got a hero's welcome, minus the crowd. John and I got to my parents' house before everyone else, to set up. The outside was illuminated by the glow of the front porch light and a single lamp somewhere inside, and we carried grocery bags containing a bottle of red wine and ingredients for a salad. My parents' neighbors had a key to the house so they could water Mom's plants; they'd hung a huge "Welcome Home" banner in the kitchen and left a plate of homemade chocolate chip cookies covered in plastic wrap on the counter. Confetti decorated the round table like fallen stars bathed in the glow of a full moon. I walked around the main floor, flicking on lights. Stephen appeared toting a pizza just as a Town Car ferrying Taylor and our parents pulled into the driveway, its high beams sweeping across the frozen lawn.

We met them in the garage. Taylor was wearing her cheetah print coat, pink scarf, and fleece hat. The dark circles under her eyes had faded, and she was smiling. Mom and Dad looked tired.

It was hard to believe my parents and Taylor had left home for Portland just one month ago. It seemed like a lifetime since John and I had flown to the West Coast for the surgery, and my sister looked so different from the little girl who had sat motionless as the hairdresser braided her long hair before cutting it short in early January.

Grandma Kathryn and Papa Jerry arrived from Raleigh the next morning. Together we painted the rock in front of The Fletcher School with purple, pink, and silver spray paint for Taylor's half-birthday. We celebrated everything those days—real birthdays and half birthdays and even dog birthdays. A cold wind blew and blurred some of the letters before the paint had dried, but Taylor didn't mind. She perched atop the rock and made funny faces for the camera. She had pink cheeks and ears and a crooked, happy expression. Her hair had already started growing back, darker than before; it covered the shiny scars on her scalp like a buzz cut.

The following day she returned to school, where she learned her girlfriends had incorporated her into their routine for the upcoming annual talent show despite her long absence. Her friend Charlotte invited her over in the afternoons to learn the words to the song they'd perform.

The night of the show, the girls wore matching t-shirts, plastic headsets, and body glitter. Taylor couldn't join her friends on the makeshift stage for safety reasons. Instead she sat offstage, singing the words to the Cheetah Girls song and snapping her fingers as the other girls performed dance moves for the families packed into the cafeteria.

While my sister and her friends went through their routine, two moms sitting behind me spoke in hushed whispers.

What was it Taylor had? Not cancer.

How much school had she missed?

How nice of the other girls to include her. She looked different since the fall; maybe it was the hair.

I shifted in my folding metal chair, which suddenly felt much more uncomfortable, and tried to tune out everything but the song. As I watched my sister chant the lyrics she'd memorized into her large plastic microphone, I saw in her an awkwardness I hadn't noticed before. I sank down in the chair as best I could, feeling sadder than I'd ever expected.

I'd thought my family would get a break after Portland. I wanted to feel grateful for the chance the surgery had given my sister. I expected to have more energy for our fundraising efforts. Except I didn't.

Taylor had survived the operation. But for the first time, she looked different from other kids. I thought of cancer patients I'd met at my hospital marketing job, people whose stories my team shared through the news media and print ads and cancer survivor calendars. As it was with many of those patients, my sister's treatment had made her look sicker. While we'd all hoped and prayed the stem cells would give her a shot, we'd known from the beginning they weren't a cure. Yet I struggled to accept everything about Portland or Taylor's illness. Maybe it's silly to wrap so much meaning into a girl's hair—one of the only things that grows back—but after they shaved my sister's head in the OR, I found I could no longer see my sister without thinking about Batten disease.

IN THE LAST days of winter, my coworker Emily, who'd helped plan the fairy tale ball fundraiser held in February, asked my parents how they felt about Taylor being a junior bridesmaid in her summer wedding.

"I can't think of anything that would make her happier," Mom said when she told me. "Of course we said yes." She and Dad worried that Taylor would have a difficult time navigating the church, but Emily had explained that her niece Hailey would also be a junior bridesmaid and could lead Taylor down the aisle.

Things hadn't been the same between Emily and me since the challenging months leading up to the fairy tale ball, when I was still getting my feet wet with fundraising, and I didn't like to think back on the event. But when I heard Emily wanted to include my sister in her big day, all I could think about was how Taylor played all of her Disney movies that included weddings until she knew every speaking part and all of the song lyrics by heart. Mom was probably right, I concluded; nothing would make my sister happier than being a junior bridesmaid in Emily's wedding.

One evening after work, Emily stopped by my parents' house to visit Taylor and share the news in person. It was an unseasonably warm night, with the faint scent of honeysuckle in the air. Emily was on her way to a meeting and didn't have time to come inside. But Taylor, always excited to greet guests, especially those who came to the house for her, ran out to visit with Emily on the front porch. They stood bathed in a disc of yellow light, talking about Taylor's favorite subjects at school and Emily's cat Snickers. After a minute Emily kneeled down and whispered something in Taylor's ear, and my sister threw her arms around the taller woman. When Taylor let go, I caught a glimpse of her face in the porch light. She was on cloud nine. Watching them together on my parents' porch that night, I loved Emily for making my sister smile. Taylor's happiness meant more to me than anything.

ONE DAY IN late March, Mom called to ask if Taylor could come to my house for a few hours while she and Dad ran an errand. I answered yes, but only if Taylor let me watch the college basketball tournament games.

"She said that's fine," Mom said. "She asked if she can bring the pompoms that go with her UNC cheerleader outfit from last Halloween and help you cheer."

A smile tugged at the corners of my lips. "Tell her to bring them."

When my parents deposited Taylor on my front porch that afternoon, she was wearing her full cheerleader outfit under her pink windbreaker, and she was clutching the light blue and white pompoms in her mitten-clad hands. Mom handed me a bag with my sister's meds and her pink case full of DVDs in the event that she got bored with the game.

We made homemade sugar cookies before tip-off. Taylor sat on the counter with her legs dangling off the side while I washed the dishes. She was eating a still-warm cookie, and she had sugar crystals on her chin.

"Laura?"

"Yes, T?" I ran a cloth under hot water and wiped crumbs into the sink.

"When I go to the Tar Heel school, will I get to be a real cheerleader?"

No, I thought. *You won't get to be a real cheerleader, and you won't ever go to the Tar Heel school. You'll be lucky to make it through high school.* My eyes darted to the drying rack in the sink stacked high with clean bowls and measuring cups. I fought the urge to throw my heavy marble rolling pin on the floor and watch it shatter into a million pieces.

I didn't tell my sister any of this. Instead, I put down the rag I was holding and wrapped her in a hug. "You can do whatever you want, sweetheart," I said. I hated lying to her, but I hated the truth more. And the truth, dark and real and burning deep inside of me, was something I thought a kid Taylor's age couldn't possibly comprehend. We couldn't hide my sister's learning difficulties or failing vision from her; she lived with those obstacles every day. But while every situation is different, my family believed telling Taylor about all of challenges to come would have been cruel. My sister didn't need to know she was facing seizures and speech loss and wheelchairs and feeding tubes, too. She didn't need to know she was dying. What could she or anyone gain from that?

ON A SUNDAY afternoon a few weeks later, John and I took Taylor to Charlotte's Discovery Place science museum, where a dinosaur exhibit was on display for several months. Discovery Place was usually a great outing for my sister, as many of its exhibits were tactile-based. But the dinosaurs and the fossils were mostly roped off and encased in glass. I watched other kids gaze up at the prehistoric creatures, their eyes big as saucers, while Taylor's sightless eyes wandered. It hadn't occurred to me that my sister, who compensated for the loss of sight with her acute hearing and sense of touch, wouldn't be able to hear or touch these exhibits. I struggled to put myself in her shoes. How could I describe the enormity of a Tyrannosaurus Rex to my sister who'd never seen one?

"The T-Rex's toe is as long as your dog, Sunny," I said. "His teeth are longer than your hand." Taylor's eyes grew wide, and her mouth formed a perfect "O." I took her wrist and led her to the plant-eating Stegosaurus. "We're standing at the tip of the Stegosaurus's tail," I told her. "Now, let's walk to his nose. Can you count your steps?" Thirty deliberate steps later, Taylor was breathless from excitement. "He's long," she agreed.

I watched as John helped Taylor with the interactive exhibits, putting his hands over hers and performing the tasks with her. She nodded when I explained that some dinosaurs ate meat, while others only ate plants, and some, like most humans, ate both. Later in the dim IMAX theater, my sister sat stick-straight on the edge of her seat, listening like there'd be a pop quiz later as two velociraptors fought to the death onscreen. Afterward in the exhibit hall, we pulled off to one side to read the museum brochure. Nearby, a crowd of kids watched a live presentation on dinosaur eggs. They laughed and clapped at all the right times; out of the corner of my eye, I saw a look of longing to be normal again wash over my sister. Her entire body froze, her head cocked in the direction of the stage as she listened, her face taut. However, when we started walking, her faraway expression disappeared, replaced with the smile she'd had all afternoon.

I know Taylor wanted to be like those kids. But she never said she wished she could be someone else, someone who didn't have to live every day systematically losing the ability to do all of the things she used to be able to do. Even on her worst days, Taylor smiled. Even on her worst days, she believed she'd beat Batten disease, even if no one else did. Whatever she may have been thinking or feeling, she never asked, *"Why me?"* She just proceeded to live her life as best she could. Taylor's resilience always amazed me.

"YOUR SISTER HAS big plans," Mom said to me on the phone not long after the afternoon at Discovery Place.

"Like what?" I asked, guessing Taylor wanted to go back to Disney World.

"Well, she wants to go to the Tar Heel school," Mom said, referring to my alma mater, UNC.

"She has good taste," I said, my heart swelling with pride.

"After that, she wants to go to vet school at N.C. State."

I smiled. "Okay. Then what?"

"After she finishes vet school, she wants to go to law school at Northwestern, like Callie."

Before heading to law school at Northwestern, my friend Callie had started sending care packages with the words "Taylor's Secret Fan Club" scrawled above the return address, and the packages hadn't stopped coming once she moved. Taylor loved ripping open the padded envelopes and catching the earrings and crayons and flavored lip balms that tumbled out.

"So . . ." my mother continued. "There's one more thing. Your sister says she's driving herself and Sunny to Chicago for law school."

I felt a pit forming in my stomach. I admired my sister's childish wonder. I wished she could be a doctor, a vet, and a lawyer. But Taylor's dream of driving the open road to Chicago with her dog beside her ripped my heart out. So she believed she'd grow up and do something normal with her life. She even expected to drive a car.

Like Taylor, I'd always been a dreamer. But all I wanted after Portland was to be like everyone else. I wanted to go to work in the morning and come home to my husband at night; I wanted to take my sister out for ice cream on the weekends and help with her homework and watch her soccer games. What I wanted, Batten disease had stolen.

A FEW DAYS before Emily's wedding, I was back at Mom and Dad's to celebrate Stephen's twenty-first birthday. Between dinner and cake, Taylor slid out of her chair and ran upstairs. A minute later, she reappeared carrying a shoebox.

"Can I practice, Mom?" She tugged the lid off and dropped it on the floor. I peered inside the box.

"Are those your shoes for the wedding, T?" I asked. The strappy sandals had a one-inch heel.

"They're my bridesmaid shoes," Taylor said, beaming. She sat down in the middle of the kitchen floor and began working at the straps.

"You can practice, T," Mom said from the sink, where she was scrubbing the remnants of homemade macaroni and cheese from a casserole dish. "Why don't you let Laura help you?"

I put my hand on my sister's and helped her undo the small buckles on the off-white slingback shoes. I guided her feet into the shoes, buckled them, and helped her stand. She looked small in her fuzzy pink Hello Kitty pajamas and heels, like a young boy who has tried on his father's suit and dress shoes.

"Heel to toe," she chanted. "Mom said heel to toe." She took one unsteady step forward, almost toppling over. I lurched to break her fall, but she righted herself and kept going. "Heel to toe." Her arms were outstretched, straight and steady; her fingertips made contact with the walls as she advanced down the narrow hallway off the kitchen. "Heel to toe." She dropped her arms to her sides. "Heel to toe." She never fell.

MOM WAS THE emotional leader of Taylor's Tale, and she'd been absent for most of the winter. But we couldn't stop working, and the steering committee met not long after she returned to Charlotte. My mother and I had all but decided we'd had enough stress for one year and didn't plan to attend the Batten Association's annual conference in July, even though we'd been in touch with the director, Lance Johnston, about extending our support of Sandy Hofmann's work at the University of Texas Southwestern.

Since the success of our early fundraisers, we'd considered applying to establish Taylor's Tale as a 501(c)(3) public charity. I appreciated and admired the Batten Association team, but I was our committee's most vocal supporter for setting up an independent, not-for-profit organization. By working through a national organization, we lost an important direct line of communication to the researchers we funded. Plus, the Batten Association had a lot of irons in the fire. It had to worry about operating costs and ice cream parties and baseball game outings at the annual conference. In my mind at least, all of that stuff equaled dollars we didn't have to end the awfulness. And I thought we could do a better job moving life-saving research forward if we made Taylor's Tale a legal entity.

Others disagreed. One of our committee members invited an attorney to our spring meeting. He explained the considerable expense and time demands required to start and run a public charity; several of the women in the room nodded in agreement, but I wasn't ready to back down. Actually, I agreed with the attorney and most of our team that we were facing an uphill battle—I just assumed we'd figure out how to climb.

By the time the trays of pimento and egg salad sandwiches and pitchers of iced tea were cleared and I had to head back to the office, we'd agreed to partner with the Batten Association to award Dr. Hofmann a second grant at its July conference. But the whole non-profit status conversation remained open, like a feather twisting in the wind.

MY FRIEND EMILY'S wedding was on the North Carolina coast in the three-hundred-year-old town of Beaufort, a land of salt marshes and wild ponies and colonial architecture. The air was thick with summer and sunblock and fried fish and young love. We checked into the inn early Friday afternoon, along with a crowd of people carting rolling suitcases and hanging dress bags.

Emily and her fiancé Greg had a large wedding party. Emily's niece Hailey, the other junior bridesmaid, was two months younger than Taylor. She had straight brown hair and an accent thick with the notes of the small towns sprinkling eastern North Carolina's coastal plains. Hailey and her little sister Bella, the flower girl, ran up and down the inn's upstairs balcony singing songs while my sister sat cross-legged and quiet on my parents' bed, listening to a movie.

I didn't have enough time to explore Beaufort when we arrived but felt as if I might suffocate within our small room's drab, wallpapered walls, so I was glad when we headed to lunch at a seafood restaurant a few blocks down the road. Emily's family thought the kids might want to sit together, so they put Hailey across from Taylor.

Blindness had made maneuvering a plate of food with a fork and spoon difficult for Taylor, and in recent months she'd taken to eating with her hands when she got frustrated. Hailey watched my sister like she had three heads, her own fork suspended over her plate of seafood. Even though Hailey was only a kid, it was all I could do not to reach over the water pitchers and platters of crab legs and shake her. *She can't help it,* I thought. *If she didn't have this godforsaken disease you two might even be friends.* Hailey avoided speaking to Taylor during dinner.

Later that afternoon when we left for the rehearsal at the town's Methodist church, Taylor looked grown-up in a black sundress with white polka dots, a white cable-knit sweater, and stud earrings that sparkled beneath her short hair.

We watched from a pew as Hailey and Taylor entered the sanctuary for their walk. Hailey stiffly took Taylor's arm as instructed and led her down one of two diagonal, thick-carpeted aisles leading to the altar.

Thinking of Taylor's school friends who fought over the privilege of walking my sister to class, I imagined Hailey would be thrilled to have such an important role. But I could see the reluctance on her face even from my seat near the front of the church.

"She doesn't want to do this," I whispered to John. "She's miserable."

My spirits lifted halfway through the rehearsal dinner at the North Carolina Aquarium when Emily made her way to our table and presented gifts to Taylor—a stuffed pony and a pink and brown purse to match her bridesmaid dress. Taylor ran her fingertips along the pony's soft mane and close-cropped coat, her sense of touch sending thousands of signals to her brain.

"What do you say, sweetheart?" Mom said.

Taylor ducked her head and smiled. "Thank you, Emily." Without letting go of the pony, she opened her arms wide and waited for a hug. Beaming, Emily kneeled down and hugged my sister. "You're welcome."

I'd had three bites of chocolate cake when the groom's college friend stood to offer a toast, his champagne glass hand unsteady. The soft murmurs throughout the room died down first to a whisper, then a dead silence as the groomsman tailspinned into a crude, sexual roast—something about wedding nights and boobs.

"Yeah, so y'all think Greg's a sweet guy," he was saying. "But he punched me in the balls just last night." He paused, looking around at the embarrassed faces of the other guests for encouragement. Someone snickered so loudly, I was sure the fish could hear it in the aquarium proper. I twisted in my chair, only to hear the laugh again. That's when I realized it had come from my sister. Still holding her stuffed pony, she had a huge grin on her face. Her eyes were cast downward, as if she were trying to hide beneath the banquet hall's bright lights.

Mom saw the grin too and laughed. Her laughter was full-throated and kindhearted, and it filled the silent room. It was the bright spot in a long, uncomfortable silence broken by the groomsman, who eventually finished his roast. The guests whooped and clapped when he ended with "Thank you," more for his conclusion than his words.

EVERYONE ELSE WAS still sleeping as I lay in the light of dawn slanting through the vertical blinds. In an hour the inn would be bustling with wedding preparations, but now the world was silent and I watched dust particles swirl in the soft sunbeams.

The weekend I got married, I had loved these moments—the secret space between events when I was alone with the world and my thoughts. I closed my eyes and remembered my solo walk along Blowing Rock's Main Street on the morning of my wedding. The sky was heavy with moisture, and the dew had settled on the park benches and the leaves of the trees. The aromas of ham biscuits at Sonny's Grill and the day's first batch of waffle cones at Kilwins had mixed with the smells of wet asphalt and clean mountain air.

I never saw my sister happier than the three days she spent in Blowing Rock to be my senior flower girl. This was a month before the Batten diagnosis brought our world crashing down. She took our cousin Morgan under her wing, showing her the proper way to hold her bouquet and clutching her hand as they descended the steep stone stairs that became our aisle when the rain moved our garden wedding indoors. When I threw my bouquet later, it had landed at Emily's feet. She bent down, picked it up, and straightened to find my sister gazing up at her. Emily wasn't engaged to Greg at the time, but she knelt down again till she and Taylor were eye-level, and she gave the bouquet to my sister. Taylor being Emily's junior bridesmaid seemed to fulfill the promise of that day.

I was still holding onto that memory hours later. By then we'd eaten our fill of croissants and fresh fruit from the inn's complimentary breakfast spread and returned to our room to play a game of musical showers, put on our wedding finery, and make the short trip back to the church for Emily and Greg's ceremony. Taylor showered first, and she sat on the edge of my parents' bed in her junior bridesmaid dress. Normally she'd be listening to a movie; instead today she strung plastic beads for a necklace, and our room was quiet except for the muffled sound of running water in the bathroom. I could hear women's voices and laughter and music next door.

"I'm going to get a soda," I said to Mom, who was applying her makeup at the mirror tacked on the closet door. "I'll be back in a minute." I had no intention of buying a soda, and I didn't bother to take my wallet when I slipped on my sandals and went outside, making sure the door shut behind me.

I walked toward the vending area on our floor. The door to the room next to ours was propped open. Inside Emily, her mom, and sister-in-law, and all of her bridesmaids, including her college friends and her nieces Hailey and Bella, were having their hair and makeup done together. A photographer darted around the room snapping pictures. The song "Carolina Girls" played from iPod speakers on the dresser.

The color started beneath the collar of the t-shirt I'd worn to breakfast. I felt it creep up my neck and into my cheeks. I turned my face away from the happy scene and continued to the vending area, where I kicked the old Pepsi machine as hard as I could, wishing I'd brought money. After a minute, I turned around and walked back empty-handed, taking care to pretend I was in too much of a hurry to say hello when I passed the hair and makeup party. After I'd shut the door to our room, I sat down on the edge of the bed next to Taylor and wrapped an arm around her. "Do you want some lip gloss for the wedding, T?"

I wasn't going to tell Mom how Taylor had been excluded, but she'd left her compact in the car and ran down to retrieve it while I was in the shower, so she saw it anyway. "I'm not telling Taylor," she said so only I could hear while I was drying my hair.

"I'm not telling either."

"It sucks," she said, her eyes filling and threatening to ruin her perfect mascara. "Batten disease sucks."

"It sucks," I agreed. "But T thinks being in this wedding is the best thing ever. So let's go have a good time."

TAYLOR'S HEEL TO toe system worked. She and Hailey made it to the front of the sanctuary and back without any falls. But the reception is what I'll always remember.

The band and the crowd fell into rhythm not long after dinner plates were cleared from the linen-covered tables. Though most of the bridesmaids were barefooted by the time the sun dipped behind the sails on the water outside, Taylor danced in her heels, clutching my wrists and dipping low to the floor, swinging her hips to the music. My sister danced like no one was watching. She clapped her hands to go along with the music or just because she was happy. Some of the anger I'd felt in the hotel room that morning melted away; as the night wore on and I had a few glasses of wine and lost my own shoes, I temporarily forgave my friend and the other women for excluding my sister.

Years have passed since Taylor's only turn as a junior bridesmaid, and I've had a lot of time to reflect. So much changed in the months between the surgery in Portland and the wedding in Beaufort. Some things were the same—her school and her teachers and her group of friends. But she took more medicine and saw doctors more often; her vision only continued to worsen, making it more obvious that she was "different," and after they shaved her head, her hair grew back darker and coarser.

Many nights I'd lie in bed, angry that my sister was sick and bitter about things that made our road tougher than it had to be. Instead of sheep I'd count the experiences she wouldn't have and the memories she'd never make. I remembered the sight of her beaming face as she walked down the aisle on Hailey's arm but could only imagine how much she would have also enjoyed the bridal party's hair and makeup session. They could have invited her, I suppose. But it was unfair to blame Emily and her family and friends for setting out to give Taylor the storybook wedding experience she wouldn't have otherwise gotten again and falling short of perfect. It took me a long time to learn that no one really knows how to handle Batten disease, even if they try.

That's where Taylor and I differed in our approach to her illness. Whether she missed various details or chose not to acknowledge them, she always focused on the good in people and situations. And so it was that when the moonlight glistened on the sound, the band stopped playing, and the single girls gathered for the bouquet toss, my sister did what any girl at a wedding would do. She found a spot at the front of the crowd. And she waited.

Chapter 8

THE MORNING AFTER the wedding, I wanted fresh air and distance from Batten disease. All at once, I felt the stress of the past three years—Taylor's early vision loss and struggles in school, the diagnosis, fundraising, Portland, the events of the weekend—closing in on me, suffocating me. Though it was no fault of theirs, I wanted to be far away from my sister and family and anything that reminded me of our new lives.

North Carolina is not large like California or Texas, but traveling from the mountains in the west to the ocean in the east can be a daunting prospect, and the only east-west interstate runs across the northern part of the state. It can take a family of four prone to frequent pit stops half a day to make the journey from my hometown of Charlotte (on the South Carolina border) to the beaches of southeastern North Carolina, less than two hundred miles as the crow flies. The beaches of the Outer Banks, a long, narrow stretch of barrier islands just off the mainland in the vast Atlantic, are even more distant.

Since we were already near the coast for the wedding, John and I had decided to extend our stay and visit the islands. John and I left Beaufort, drove for an hour, and caught a slow-moving ferry bound for Ocracoke Island on the Outer Banks' southernmost tip. When we exited the ferry and pulled onto Highway 12, the single major road linking the islands, I asked John to stop at the first public beach access. Before he turned off the engine I opened my car door and bounded onto the wild beach. Stopping short of the surf, I dug my heels into the sand and felt the afternoon breeze whip through my hair.

I didn't realize I'd closed my eyes until John wrapped his arms around me.

"What are you thinking about?" His voice was soft, yet it pierced the silence.

"I'm not thinking about anything," I said. That was true. My mind was blank, like the deserted seashore. I watched a single seagull land in the wet sand glistening in the sunlight near the high tide line. I noticed other sets of tiny seagull tracks, looping in and out of the water in crooked lines and zigzags and makeshift figure eights. Some of them disappeared into the ocean. A second bird landed nearby while we stood watching the first, its white feathers stark against the dark sand. The wind strengthened, and the long grasses on the dunes bobbed and swayed. Things that had worried me drifted away on the salt breeze.

In that instant it was tempting to set up permanent residence on the island—a full day's drive from Charlotte, with spotty Internet and wireless service. It wasn't the first time I'd imagined wiping the slate clean. Maybe it would have been easier to let it all wash away, gone forever, like sandcastles at the changing of the tide.

But if I'd done that, a large part of me would have been lost forever, too.

While on the Outer Banks that week, John and I visited Jockey's Ridge, the largest living sand dune on the East Coast. The Carolina sun hung high in the clear blue sky, and the deep sand blazed beneath our bare feet. For hours we made a point of finding the tallest, steepest sand hills, standing at the crest, joining hands, closing our eyes, and running to the bottom as fast as we could. In those moments I wished Taylor was with us, because flying down those hills would have given her so much joy.

Deep down I knew I couldn't forget my sister or her illness, no matter how many highway miles or ferry rides I put between us; I couldn't leave the people I loved to fight our battle alone. And one week after landing on Ocracoke Island's deserted southern shore, I did what I'd always known I'd do. I drove home with John, and I started fighting again.

IT WAS JULY—the month of fireworks and lightning bugs and the anniversary of Taylor's diagnosis. As planned, Mom and I stayed home when other families and scientists convened for the Batten Association's annual conference, but our committee sent the Association a check for $55,000 to extend Dr. Hofmann's research on infantile Batten disease for twelve months. It was nice waging war against Batten disease from a distance, without the added emotional burden of seeing all those affected kids at the conference. Taylor hadn't had the easiest of years, and

Portland had changed her forever, but she was still talking and walking. Compared to a lot of Batten kids she was the picture of health, and in those days I wasn't strong enough to spend days in a cramped hotel with all of those crystal balls.

Meanwhile, I hadn't given up on establishing Taylor's Tale as a public charity, despite the attorney's cautionary tale and general reluctance among our committee members. I cornered Mom near the end of a long walk in her neighborhood after dinner one night.

"Have you thought any more about our 501(c)(3) talk?"

Mom didn't look my way, but her gait slowed. I turned to gaze at her. We had just crossed onto her street and were passing beneath a streetlamp. Framed by its radiant light in the midst of the darkness, her profile glowed. She looked like a superhero.

"Yes."

"And what have you decided?"

"I haven't decided." But she lingered on the words.

"I think you have."

Mom stopped walking, right at the edge of the streetlamp's disc of light. She twisted and looked right at me. The world beyond the lamplight faded to black. We were all alone, in a moment suspended in time. Somehow I knew that the future of Taylor's Tale hung in the balance.

"I want to be in control of my own destiny," my mother said, her voice barely above a whisper. Even today I'm still not sure if she was talking to the stars or to me. "This is life or death, right? If we're meant to fail, we'll fail. But I want it to be on us."

"So we fight it head-on," I said, emboldened, my voice rising on the quiet street. "We could keep doing what we're doing. We might make some headway. But we could focus one hundred percent on funding the science that can save kids like T. Don't you want to change the world?"

Gone were all the questions I'd previously asked myself. *What would it take to cure Batten disease? How long would it take? How would we do it? Who would help us?* I didn't ask myself if it was crazy to believe we could sustain our early success. We'd raised money in our own community, from our friends who felt moved by our story, but I didn't question whether we could grow beyond our hometown. I didn't wonder about the five hundred-odd American kids—maybe less than a few thousand in the whole world—with Batten disease who maybe could be cured by research we funded.

Instead, on that hot summer night, days removed from the two-year anniversary of the worst day of our lives, I was confident. Hope wasn't a strong enough word for how I felt about our chances to succeed on our own. I *believed*. I was twenty-six years old. I didn't have any non-profit experience or know-how except for the few fundraisers we'd held, not all of which had gone off without a hitch. I didn't know the first thing about the legal issues associated with starting a public charity. I just knew it felt right.

Suddenly, I heard my mother saying yes, she wanted to change the world, and she believed in Taylor's Tale, too.

MARTHA, OUR STEERING committee chair, agreed to serve as the first president of our new board. A local law firm prepared our 501(c)(3) paperwork and submitted it to the IRS. And in late August, a few days after Taylor's tenth birthday, Taylor's Tale became a public charity. I announced the news on my blog.

The board looked a lot like the steering committee that had raised well over $100,000 for the Batten Association. It was stocked with volunteers extraordinaire, past presidents of Junior Leagues and symphonies and community councils, all trained to tackle a cause. It was a volunteer dream team primed—on paper at least—to kick Batten's ass.

But even in the charity's infancy I could tell the recent fairy tale ball discord had changed our group. There was an irreparable divide between the old guard and the new guard, and looking back now, I think a lot of our original committee members stuck around more out of respect for my mom than because they believed we could beat Batten disease. However, in those days I had an unshakable trust in anyone who claimed to be an ally. I'd defend my values like my life depended on it, but at the end of the day I *wanted* to believe in people. And even if friends let me down, I wanted to believe they had our best interests at heart. Saving Taylor meant everything to me, and sometimes that single-minded focus caused me to miss important signs.

AROUND THE TIME we filed the paperwork for Taylor's Tale, my sister brought some paperwork of her own home from school. A week or so after she started her fifth grade year at Fletcher, she informed my parents she was signing up for Girls on the Run, a youth development program that includes training for a 5K race.

Mom called me to check in and casually mentioned that Taylor had joined the team.

"How can she run a 5K if she's blind?" I asked even as I smiled, not at all surprised. "How is that safe?"

"We'll figure it out," she said. She didn't sound concerned. "I'm supposed to call Martha about our first board meeting in a few minutes. Don't worry about your sister; she always finds a way."

A few days later, Taylor—and The Fletcher School—found a way in the shape of seventeen-year-old Mary-Kate Behnke. A student in the upper school, Mary-Kate said sure, she'd stay after school in the afternoons to be Taylor's running buddy.

In early September, Taylor and her girlfriends and Mary-Kate started practice. Coach Diane, the lower school counselor, and Coach Cathy, a community volunteer, taught the fifth graders about things like good fitness habits, teamwork, and self-esteem. After their lessons, the girls walked or ran laps around the track. Taylor and Mary-Kate each held one end of a shortened jump rope—my sister's lifeline.

Taylor threw herself into the team. She led cheers and laughed off the sticky heat that lingered well into autumn. "She was the life of the party," her friend Charlotte told me years later. "She made practice fun." My sister shook off bruised elbows and scraped knees on the days she fell, the victim of a simple errant pebble or an untied shoelace or just plain being blind.

Meanwhile, I threw myself into Taylor's Tale. I blogged several times a week and revamped our website; I helped put on small fundraisers and kept up with researchers around the world. I started running more to manage the stress. Physical activity had always been an outlet for me, but that fall it took on new meaning. Running through a tunnel of trees and breathing fresh air had a calming effect, and I could always count on a runner's high—that moment when happy chemicals called endorphins flowed into my brain and I believed I could overcome everything we were fighting. On particularly beautiful days I tried to imagine my sister's experience as a blind runner. Once I even closed my eyes and tried to run in a straight line. Within a few seconds I felt the concrete sidewalk change to grass as I veered off course, and I opened my eyes just in time to dodge a telephone pole. I kept my eyes open the rest of the way.

Of course, I'd never been as brave as my little sister. Just that summer on our annual trip to the beach, Taylor had run from our lounge chairs to the ocean and back again without our assistance. She may have been going blind, but she had one hell of an internal compass, and she had no fear.

I still have a photo of Taylor walking around the Fletcher track with Mary-Kate at a Girls on the Run practice. Her hair had gotten longer over the summer, and even though she was only ten it was obvious she'd have a cute figure someday. In the picture, she's wearing a fitted t-shirt and short cotton shorts, and her legs are long and slender. She's not looking at the camera, but it's impossible to tell she's blind except for the fact that she and Mary-Kate are tethered by a jump rope. She doesn't look like the kids with leukemia or congenital heart defects who were patients at the hospital where I worked. She doesn't look like she's dying.

On the surface, my sister had a lot in common with her classmates in those days, but still people who knew about the disease would gesture toward her and whisper, "How long?" Though they meant well, I always hated that question. Why did I have to give my sister an expiration date? Kids like Taylor were all so different and there were so few that generalizations didn't apply, and anyway we weren't going to get to that point. We were going to save T, and we were going to savor each day in the process.

IN EARLY OCTOBER the sky fell. My Grandma Kathryn slipped outside her beauty shop in Raleigh and broke her hip. I'm not sure what most families would have done, but we dropped everything and drove to Raleigh, even though it was the middle of the week. Mom cancelled a Taylor's Tale meeting, and for once I didn't update my blog.

While she was in the hospital my grandmother had vivid hallucinations and acted out dreams, even baking a cake—cracking eggs and all. She was diagnosed with a brain disease called Lewy body dementia, and we moved her to a hospital in Greensboro closer to Uncle David. A surgeon there performed a total hip replacement, and a neurologist on staff told us all of the awful things about her disease—things we'd already heard from David because he was a brain doctor.

I burned up the hundred miles of highway between my house and the hospital that month, often driving north to visit my grandmother after work and returning home late that night. Watching her sleep, I had a lot of time to reflect, and after the initial shock had worn off, I acknowledged the subtle warning signs we'd attributed to depression stemming from T's illness and my uncle Mike's recent heart attack. *We missed so much,* I told myself, a thought eerily similar to the one that ran through my head in the early days after Taylor's diagnosis. But of course it was too late and there was only so much we could do.

One night, I sat alone in the hospital room in Greensboro and tried to imagine that the woman in the bed with the drawn face and uncombed hair was my grandmother. Grandma Kathryn had helped me find sand dollars on the Oak Island shore and write poetry while driving on the interstate in eastern North Carolina; together, we found beauty in a scrubby patch of wildflowers perched on a hill and the contrails of jets, like giant white crayons drawing lines in the sky. We hung an old sheet in the windows of her house and played cards in our pajamas or watched stacks of movies on the sofa bed until after midnight in the summer. She had always been my closest confidante, and in that moment it hit me that I was facing the possibility of losing my sister without my grandmother beside me.

Grandma Kathryn went home on Halloween, her birthday. I waited for her life to normalize—for things to get back to some semblance of the way they were before. But she was never the same.

Brain disease really is a bitch. But looking back, even I was guilty of letting brain disease win sometimes when I should have fought harder. When Grandma Kathryn gestured to her dogs flopped in front of the fireplace even though she hadn't had a dog for years, I got frustrated, not with my grandmother but with the shapeless monster stealing her from me.

"They've been out in the yard and they're tired now," she'd say, pointing at a spot on the Oriental rug. "I love my little dogs."

"What dogs?" I'd ask. "There aren't any dogs here." She wouldn't respond, but her eyes would fill and plead for understanding. I thought telling her the truth was the kind thing to do, but it only made her sadder and more confused.

When Lewy body dementia affected her cognitive skills, I sometimes addressed my grandmother like a child. When it attacked her emotions, leading to spontaneous crying spells, I didn't do enough to make her feel better; mostly I just cried, too.

I wasn't wired to handle my grandmother's illness; it struck too quickly and too fully, and I wasn't prepared to give her the love and support she deserved. I understand now that in the absence of one skill or tool, we often compensate in other ways. My sister taught me a lot about that. Just that fall she'd finished learning braille in less than a year. "I made it to Z!" she announced when I came over to visit one night, running down the stairs clutching a worksheet filled with the raised dots of the braille alphabet. She led me into the kitchen where her braille typewriter was set up and showed me how she could type words like "zebra" and "zoo." I hugged her and tried to remember if I'd ever gotten that excited about homework.

IN THE MIDDLE of dealing with my grandmother's accident and subsequent diagnosis and getting the pieces of our fledgling charity in order, autumn came and went. Before I knew it, the nights were cold again and the mall was decorated for Christmas.

Taylor's Girls on the Run season finished on a frigid morning in early December at uptown Charlotte's Thunder Road 5K. John and I pulled into Mom and Dad's driveway just as a dull orange glow lit the inky sky. On the floor of her room upstairs, my sister silently tugged on athletic pants and thick socks, her exposed skin dotted with goose bumps. She was wearing her blue team shirt over a hot pink fleece pullover. I helped her pin her race bib onto her t-shirt and tie her running shoes.

"You're going to do awesome, T," I said to get her talking. She didn't respond, and the look on her face was hard to interpret. Taylor had loved everything about this experience. Yet here she was, getting ready for her big day, and I couldn't get a peep out of her. I wanted so badly to read her mind right then—to understand what she was going through—but

I couldn't, and I didn't ask. I wasn't sure if we'd shared a private moment or if she'd drifted into a world I could never fully comprehend.

In the kitchen downstairs, she was back to her usual self. When Mary-Kate arrived, Taylor sang her name. She sang between clicks as we took group photos with the huge Fletcher School sign the coaches would carry during the race; we'd painted it with candy canes and Christmas lights the previous night. She sang along to Christmas carols from the third row of my SUV starting the moment we pulled out of the neighborhood until I squeezed into a too-small parking space in the crush of runners uptown.

It wasn't until we climbed out of the car that we discovered the jump rope Mary-Kate had used to guide Taylor all season was missing. I felt a weird sensation deep in my gut. *There's no way Taylor and Mary-Kate can run a 5K in that crowd without the jump rope*, I thought.

I should have known not to doubt my sister.

The bungee cord, stowed in the back of my car for a rainy day, was John's idea. Though not perfect, it was about the same length as the jump rope. The girls held it as we headed for the start line. I watched as Taylor grew used to the feel of the bungee cord's unfamiliar hook in the palm of her hand, running her fingertips over its curves and lines as we walked and making a fist over the cord when we stopped for traffic.

My sister may have been the only blind person running that day, but thousands take part in the annual marathon, half marathon, and 5K. The crowd engulfed us as we approached the start line. When we arrived in the heart of uptown Charlotte, we ducked inside the warm convention center to join Taylor's teammates and coaches. The moment we found them, my sister's friends surrounded her. A smile spread across her face as their voices reached her ears. When Coach Diane and Coach Cathy took the train of girls back out into the cold for the start of the race minutes later, Taylor led them all in song, their notes lingering as fine, white puffs in the December air. And then, they were running, the fuzzy white ball of Taylor's Santa hat bouncing in time against the clear blue sky.

The throng of mostly taller runners quickly swallowed my sister, but at first I tracked her and Mary-Kate by following the Fletcher team sign as it bobbed above the crowd. Soon, even that became impossible, so I drifted toward the finish area, and I waited. I tugged my toboggan down over my ears, and I tried to stay warm.

Fifty-three minutes later, I was still shivering in the cold sunshine when Taylor crossed the finish line with her running buddy, her fingers curled around the bungee cord, her face turned toward heaven.

I'd spent so much of the past two-plus years focusing on the ugliness of Batten disease. But when Taylor and Mary-Kate crossed the finish line together, there was nothing ugly about that moment. Whereas I'd often felt only anger toward Batten disease, my sister had beaten her demons by ignoring them—by focusing not on what she'd lost, but on what she could still do. She didn't waste her time worrying about what Batten disease had taken from her. She paid it no mind, and she ran her race.

Before the trees bloomed in the spring, I'd started running for her.

Chapter 9

IN THOSE WINTER months after Taylor's race, I ran like my life depended on it; in truth maybe it did. And for the first time, I was running for something greater than myself.

I liked setting out from my driveway without a predetermined route, running along the South Charlotte streets I'd driven for ten years and seeing them from a new perspective, watching other people live their lives and getting lost in my own head. I liked feeling the crunch of frozen pine needles underneath the soles of my shoes and the dry, cold air as it flowed into my lungs. I felt alive.

Taylor's achievement as a runner had awakened something in me. Though I'd played soccer in college, I was now in the best shape of my life. I ran all the time. The endorphins made me feel powerful—invincible even. They were like a drug and I was addicted.

Not long after the holidays, I put my addiction to good use and signed up to run my first race in Taylor's honor: the half marathon at Thunder Road, still ten months away. My sister's courage as a blind runner had resonated with people, and I'd convinced myself I had to fight Batten disease through the sport. I hadn't quite figured how all the dots connected back then, but I assumed it'd come to me one day.

Between running and Taylor's Tale work and my job, I tried really hard to spend quality time with my sister. I tried to pretend that things would never change, that she would always be able to walk through stores with me and talk to me and sing to her favorite songs in my car and perhaps even run future races with me. But deep down I knew better.

ONE NIGHT AFTER leaving the gym, I drove to my parents' house and ran up the basement steps two at a time, calling for Taylor.

"Hey, Sissy," she answered from the kitchen table upstairs, where she was working on braille homework. I heard sounds of a shower upstairs, and Mom was nowhere in sight. However, my father was asleep in the family room, that morning's newspaper and an empty coffee cup in a heap on his lap. I shook him awake. Would it be okay if I kidnapped Taylor for an hour? Dad said T had already had dinner, and he was sure it'd be fine as long as we were back in an hour.

Taylor climbed into the back seat of my car with a silly, happy grin, her cheeks already pink from the cold. "Where are we going?"

"We need to buy Daisy a birthday present," I said over my shoulder. "Then you can help me choose party decorations."

"Yessss!" She grinned and laughed and clapped her hands. "I love Daisy so much. She's such a cute puppy. I love her."

I'd never celebrated a dog's birthday before, but Taylor made it fun. We went to an expensive, boutique pet store, where she chose a hoodie with a leash hole for my dog to wear for walks on chilly nights. Next we headed to Party City, where I dropped forty dollars on dog-themed decorations and favors for the party and a charm bracelet for Taylor. She sang songs and skipped down the aisles, only once crashing into a cart someone had left unattended.

On the short drive back to my parents' house I asked her about school. Did she like her classes? When was the next talent show?

"My teachers said I'm not going to do math anymore," she told me. "I'm not good at it." Without warning, the mood in the car shifted. It was palpable. Even the radio switched to a sad song. It was a clear night and stars dotted the sky, but I flashed back to that rainy afternoon at Starbucks when simple number problems drove my six-year-old sister to cry. It felt like a lifetime ago . . . yet here we were, Batten's earliest symptoms coming to bear, and the worst still to come.

I dropped off my sister two minutes after eight p.m., just in time for her to get ready for school the next day. She stood at the front window, clutching her new charm bracelet and waving goodbye.

The five-minute drive home gave me way too much time to think. By the time I pulled into my driveway, I was afraid I'd put my fist through a wall if I didn't clear my head. So instead of going into the house I went for a run outside, even though I'd already completed a hard workout earlier that night and the temperature was still dropping.

I was angry at Batten disease for making Taylor feel incompetent at school. Angry at the world for harboring a monster like Batten disease. Overwhelmed by my love for my sister. In the darkness my heart pounded so hard that I half-expected to hear it between the slap, slap of my shoes against the pavement. In spite of the cold night I sweated, the droplets mixing with tears as I ran.

MY MOTHER HAD been spending a lot of time in Raleigh since Grandma Kathryn's accident and Lewy body dementia diagnosis. We'd decided it was best to move my grandparents to Greensboro where my Uncle David and Aunt Holly could look after them, but it was upsetting for everyone, and my grandmother in particular wasn't adjusting well to the stacks of packing boxes in her house and hushed conversations about her condition. Mom supported the family in ways I couldn't even fathom considering Taylor's illness and our demanding non-profit work. She helped David and Holly quarterback the situation and lent my grandmother the emotional support the rest of us couldn't muster. Some days I watched her and swore she'd cloned herself; how else could she accomplish it all without breaking under the pressure?

In late February, Mom flew to San Diego to represent Taylor's Tale at the Lysosomal Disease Network World Symposium, the same event she and Dad had attended in Orlando a few months after my sister's diagnosis. She came back with a binder full of notes and new contacts.

There were never many parents at the scientific meetings. I always found it funny that my mother, a piano major in college, ended up rubbing elbows with scientists at all those conferences. But that was how Mom reacted to her youngest child being diagnosed with a rare disease with no known cure. She ventured outside her comfort zone and fought like hell, even when some people thought she didn't belong.

While on the West Coast, Mom finally met Daniel Kerner and his mother, Joanna, who lived outside Los Angeles. Daniel and Taylor shared a special bond because they represented the bookends of the six-patient stem cell trial. In spite of my sister's long stay in Portland for the surgery and frequent return trips during the twelve-month follow-up period, our families had never crossed paths, but we'd stayed in close touch via phone and computers. Even though we'd never before met, I felt as close to the Kerners as I did to any family fighting Batten disease.

Daniel could sing and talk in complete sentences by age two, but Batten disease later stole his speech and motor skills. He went to all of his brother David's baseball games and loved Buzz Lightyear from the movie *Toy Story;* he skied down Mammoth Mountain with the help of a ski instructor and special equipment.

After his surgery in late 2006, Daniel said "Dad" for the first time in two years. But in the past several months his condition had taken a sudden turn for the worse. I'd never really believed the stem cells were a cure, but I wasn't prepared for the world to lose Daniel. I kept telling myself I'd find time to visit him in California.

Mom and Joanna exchanged gifts for the kids in San Diego: a Carolina baseball cap signed by the women's basketball coach for Daniel, and a book in braille called *Love* for Taylor.

That week, Joanna wrote about the experience on her blog. *"There is a special bond the moms share that is on a level deeper than any peer friendships. We are woven together into a different cloth of life that creates a strong and passionate quilt, assembled painfully through heartbreak and upheaval, grief and acceptance, strength and perseverance. A quilt, we hope, big and strong enough to smother the dragon and deliver our children back to their childhood dreams."*

On the other end of the continent, I wrote a letter to Daniel and published a blog about our mothers' meeting. I organized a spring fundraiser and ran five days a week. I fought the dragon.

A FEW WEEKS after Mom returned from San Diego, she and I took Taylor to my paternal grandparents' condo on South Carolina's Grand Strand for a girls-only spring break trip.

My Granddaddy Parks—my father's father—had loved this part of the coast for its golf courses and restaurants. He never spent much time on the beach, preferring to play nine holes, have lunch at the golfer Greg Norman's restaurant, play the back nine, and finish the day with dinner out on the town. Granddaddy passed away before Taylor was born, but we held on to the beach place even after Grandma Margaret's Alzheimer's got so advanced she couldn't leave her assisted living home.

The overdeveloped town bordered on tacky and had never been my kind of place, but the beach had saltwater and sand, and after twenty-four hours I was a changed person. We'd make it down to the water by late morning and often just sit in our chairs, watching the ocean with our toes in the cool sand. When our joints got stiff, we'd stand up and play catch with a soft rubber ball. You wouldn't have known Taylor was blind to watch her play. She'd set her bare feet in the soft sand, her legs squared and her knees slightly bent, like she was a first baseman waiting for a throw. Her hair, thick and full and darker than ever, fell in tousled waves across her forehead, framing gorgeous brown eyes. "It's coming to you, T," we'd say just before letting the ball fly; on cue she'd cup her arms to receive the ball. Mom and I never stopped talking, and Taylor located us by the sound of our voices, returning a perfect toss every time.

Though I'd packed enough clothes to stay for weeks, I'd forgotten some key items and decided to walk to the drugstore up the road one afternoon not long after we arrived.

"Mind if we tag along?" Mom said. "I haven't had a walk today."

"Sure," I answered. "Hey Taylor," I called toward the general direction of the kitchen, where my sister was writing "I love you" notes to her dog Sunny in an uneven hand with a fat crayon. "Let's walk to the store. You can have a special pick."

At the drugstore we perused the aisles like three girlfriends, discussing the merits of Maybelline versus L'Oreal mascara and ways to get my feet, battered by Charlotte soccer leagues and half marathon training, sandal-ready for summer. Taylor decided she needed new lip-gloss to carry in her purse. We hadn't made it back to the condo before my sister had torn into the plastic packaging and applied her cherry-flavored lip-gloss.

"At least you got one girly daughter," I said to Mom, who was laughing.

Later that night, when I'd retreated to the sofa to watch college basketball and my mother and Taylor had spread books and papers across the kitchen table to work on an upcoming school presentation, I could barely imagine that my sister was fatally ill. I lived in constant fear of the future, but the simple fun we'd found together that week was a tantalizing reminder of not only what *could* have been, but also what *was*. There were so many things I wanted to do with Taylor—take her to Hawaii, return to Disney World, see her music idols the Jonas Brothers on their world tour. But time and again she taught me about the simple joys, like our game of catch and our shopping trip to the drugstore.

Taylor was growing up; lately she'd shunned children's clothing stores in favor of brands more popular with pre-teens, like Justice and

Abercrombie & Fitch. She and her friends had officially discovered boys, too. That spring she'd carried a scrap of paper with a phone number and the words "Scott's Home Phone" around in her pocket for three days.

Of course, watching my sister discover boys and get excited over lipgloss and makeup had a catch. These changes were normal for any preteen girl, but they also signaled the passage of time—a scary prospect for a family like mine. Because we all knew what the future held for Taylor if Taylor's Tale ran out of time.

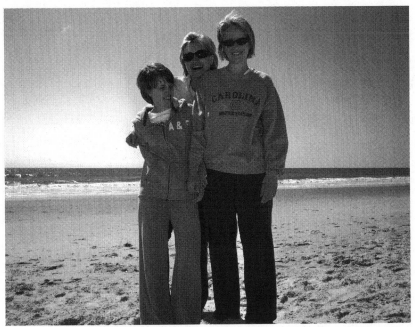

Taylor, Sharon, and Laura on the beach, 2009

I CAUGHT THE spring cleaning bug the weekend after the beach trip. After filing tax receipts and dusting ceilings and organizing desk drawers, I sat on the floor of our bedroom closet, sorting a mountain of clothes destined for the out-of-season box and donation run. I'd come home to a chaotic work schedule and busy nights, and rest hadn't come easily. Thumbing through stacks of folded t-shirts, I thought about catching up on marketing projects at the hospital and developing a new website for Taylor's Tale, as we'd outgrown the one I built on a rainy Saturday just months after the diagnosis.

It took me a moment to notice the stain. The watery black smear hovered just below the right shoulder on the white t-shirt—mascara I wasn't able to wash out after John held me the day Taylor was diagnosed with Batten disease. Seeing that black spot brought memories rushing back. Somehow we'd both squeezed into one of our hand-me-down dining room chairs; Daisy watched us from across the room, certain something was wrong. The meager dinner we'd cooked with our nice pots and pans and utensils—mostly wedding gifts so new I hadn't yet had time to write thank yous—sat uneaten on the borrowed table.

Suddenly I didn't want the shirt in my house. I flung it into the "donate" pile, face down to hide the stain.

I thought that act gave me power. But when I carried one of the out-of-season boxes to our little-used guest room a few minutes later, I caught sight of the teddy bear Taylor and I had built together that awful day. I wanted to be invincible, but I wasn't. Instead I stood alone in the middle of the room and listened to fat drops of spring rain pelt the window and cried again.

My phone rang hours later just as the rain ended. As I picked up the receiver and heard my sister's voice on the line, I saw a rainbow hanging above the treetops, like God had put it there.

AT THE END of April a family friend gave us passes to opening weekend festivities at the Great Wolf Lodge. An over-the-top family resort, it had a water park, arcade, and kids' spa with banana split sundae thrones, sherbet facial scrubs, and seventy-five dollar mani/pedis. Stephen had a few days before final exams and joined us; he and John helped Taylor win piles of tickets playing Skeeball and Whac-A-Mole. My sister squealed the loudest of anyone on the water park's giant, kaleidoscope-shaped slide; when we reached the bottom, Stephen's arms were covered in tiny white marks where she'd dug her fingernails into his skin. Then Taylor and Dad stood under a giant bucket that dumped hundreds of gallons of water on the splash play area every few minutes. Taylor wrapped her arms around Dad in a death grip and jumped up and down like she couldn't stand it, but she laughed hysterically every time they got drenched.

On Friday night, teen pop singer Mitchel Musso, from the Disney Channel's *Hannah Montana*, performed a private concert in the resort's lobby. When the music began, everyone in the crowd got on their feet, but Taylor stayed on the floor. I knelt down to within inches of her ear.

"T, do you want to get up and dance? The concert's starting." But she didn't turn toward me or make a move to stand or show any sign that she'd heard me at all. She was captivated by the sounds coming from the stage, lost in her own secret, happy little world of music. Smiling, I put down my bag and sat on the floor next to her for the rest of the show. I didn't even care that I only saw the faded jeans of the dad in front of us for an hour-plus.

As I took in the shrieks of the other preteen and tween girls while my sister sat silently, mesmerized by the music, I thought back to my own fifth grade year. I considered how hard it must be for a girl Taylor's age to endure everything she'd had to endure. Getting a rotten diagnosis. Taking nasty medicine that made her breath smell and came only in capsules so huge they hurt to swallow. Struggling to understand math and playful sarcasm. Traveling hundreds or thousands of miles for doctor visits and major surgery. Getting holes drilled into her head. Giving up her long blonde hair. Going blind.

I remembered fifth grade as the year when everything began changing for my classmates and me. Some of the girls started puberty, most of us had our first real crushes on boys, and all of us started caring about what other kids thought. All of those physical and emotional and social changes triggered the "mean girls" syndrome. That year, for the first time, kids in my class really got teased.

Thankfully Taylor hadn't been teased at school. I thought about how my sister had faced every day—every wound, every obstacle, every setback—with courage and grace. And I always thought the kids in her class probably respected her for that, even if they didn't know what to call their feelings.

All I had wanted at Taylor's age was to be like everyone else. She couldn't have that. Even Portland hadn't given her that. But she was still a ten-year-old girl who asked Mom and Dad to circle Disney movie and CD release dates on the calendar. Who lived life to the fullest despite the awful cards in her hand. Her disease made her different, but she wasn't afraid to wait in a long line to talk to the pop star Mitchel Musso at the autograph session following the concert. And like any other smitten ten-year-old girl, she refused to wash her hand in our hotel room later that night, because Mitchel had held it when they met.

ON MOTHER'S DAY weekend Taylor ran her second race with her Girls on the Run team and her running buddy, Mary-Kate. The day dawned clear and warm, and the historic neighborhood park hosting the race was awash with lush green leaves and fiery pink azaleas.

Dad and the boys played the role of faithful cheerleaders and waited at the finish line, but Mom and I wore race bibs pinned to our shirts and speed-walked behind the team. I kept one eye on them and one eye on the pavement, certain I'd fall in the stampede of girls. Taylor gripped her end of the tether and didn't let go. Her thick hair bobbed as she ran; it was dark—even in the sunlight slanting through the trees—and streaked with hot pink hairspray. All of her teammates had signed the back of her t-shirt. Out of the blue I wondered if she'd signed theirs.

"Are they going too fast?" Mom said at the first mile marker.

I shook my head. "T's fine." I jogged in front of my sister, flanked by Mary-Kate and Coach Diane, and took a few photos. Taylor was laughing; she didn't look tired.

Near the end of the race the girls came to such an abrupt stop we almost barreled into them.

"What's wrong?" my mother asked, immediately shifting into Mom mode.

I peered over Mary-Kate's shoulder and shook my head. "Nothing. Look." Someone had written the word "Believe" in chalk on the asphalt. The huge, white letters stretched across the street, and somehow the horde of runners and walkers had parted at just the right moment, like the Red Sea for Moses.

We stood there quietly, others continuing toward the finish line on either side of us. Taylor gazed in the direction of the letters inscribed on the pavement as if she could see them. That whole morning she'd been laughing and smiling and singing, but right then she had that look on her face she got sometimes, like she was miles away. And then, just like that, she started running again, tugging Mary-Kate along with her. Mom and Coach Diane and I followed. A few turns later my sister crossed the finish line, beating her previous 5K time by twelve minutes.

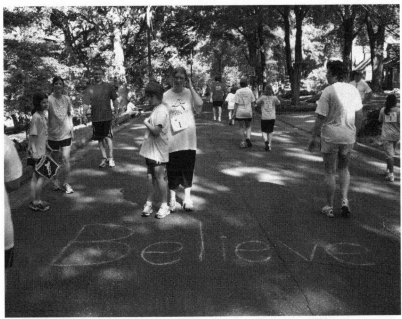

A message of hope near the end of Taylor's second 5K race, 2009

THE WHOLE NEXT month I had as much energy as I'd ever had. I'd recently launched a new blog, and after Taylor's race I worked with the hospital's creative agency to build a new website for Taylor's Tale, mapping out the pages and writing the copy. I'd gotten a promotion in January and relished a new challenge not related to Batten disease. Despite rising temperatures, I continued increasing my mileage in training for my own race. Thunder Road was still more than six months away, but I couldn't wait to run my first half marathon for my sister.

Meanwhile, Taylor needed a new doctor. Dr. Krystyna Wisniewski, the infantile Batten disease expert whose Staten Island office had been a frequent destination for my family over the past few years, had passed away in the fall. On a recommendation from our friends Chris and Wendy Hawkins, Mom and Dad took my sister to a neurologist at Duke

University Hospital. He didn't have the late Dr. Wisniewski's unique charm, but he was less than a three-hour drive from home and close to my ailing grandmother.

A few weeks after the 5K, Mom pulled Taylor out of school for a few days for a battery of tests at Duke, including her third MRI in five months and exhaustive neuropsychiatric testing. I called Mom after the second and final day to see how my sister was holding up.

"What? She's fine," Mom said, sounding distracted. Then I heard the garbled sounds of a fast food employee's voice crackling over a drive-thru window speaker. I waited for Mom to order Taylor's chicken nuggets and diet soda.

"How did the tests go? I take it you're on the way home?"

"There were a lot of tests and they were long but they were fine. We don't have any results yet. Your sister is tired but fine. Happy to be done. When we got to the car she yelled, 'Woo hoo!'"

I was so intent on picturing Taylor's celebratory moment that I forgot to respond.

"Are you still there? Do you want to talk to her? Here, she doesn't have her food yet."

"Hey, Sissy!"

"Hey T," I said. "You alright?"

"I'm done. The nurse was nice. But they put gook in my hair to hold the wires. Mom let me use her fruity shampoo."

"So your hair's clean now?" I asked, smiling.

"Yep! Can I eat now?"

"Sure. Give the phone back to Mom. I love you."

"Love you!"

"Hey," my mother said, after taking the phone from Taylor. "If you talk to your father, tell him we'll be home in two hours. He didn't pick up and his voicemail's full."

"Okay. So they put gook in her hair?"

"Yes, for the EEG. I knew about it ahead of time. I also knew she wouldn't stand to have that stuff in her hair for the car ride home. So I requested a late checkout at the hotel. She has clean, blow-dried hair and chicken nuggets and she's happy."

MOM FLEW TO Germany at the beginning of June for her second NCL Congress, the same meeting we'd attended in Rochester two years before. Like at the World Symposium in San Diego, she was a lone wolf, because she was a parent attending a scientific conference.

My mother had promised to send me daily updates. I was standing at my front window, watching the sun dip below the tops of the trees, when the first email popped into my inbox. It was after two a.m. in Hamburg, but it didn't surprise me that Mom was still awake. During a busy first day she'd met three other families: a father named Tracy whose son had been diagnosed just weeks earlier, a German family who, like us, had started a charity to fight Batten disease, and another father whose son was also in the Portland trial. That night she was hunting down scientists in the hotel bar when most people had gone out to explore the city.

I think I understood we'd entered a new world—not by choice—the first time I attended the NCL Congress with Mom in Rochester. There we were—an English major and a piano performance major—in a hotel banquet hall far from home, listening to a scientist from Washington University School of Medicine discuss the systemic and metabolic abnormalities associated with infantile neuronal ceroid lipofuscinosis— and actually understanding some of it. That was the reality of fighting an ultra-rare disease, I'd realized. You had to be willing to step outside your comfort zone and learn something new. You had to be ready to fight for yourself in case no one else would. I think those other families in Hamburg recognized that, too. Otherwise they wouldn't have been there.

Mom met and talked with researchers from the U.S., U.K., Belgium, Finland, Denmark, and Germany that first day at the conference. *During the first lunch meeting, the woman sitting next to me was from Moscow,* Mom said in her email. *We struggled with the language barrier but managed to communicate.* She heard a talk by Dr. Hofmann and learned that the work we'd funded for nearly two years was ready for preclinical testing. *She's made the enzyme; now she has to figure out how to get it to the brain.* As Mom faithfully sent updates, I shared them in a series of blog posts about the Congress.

The final session was a moment my mother both craved and feared, as the results of the Portland stem cell trial would be shared publicly for the first time. We knew Taylor was still declining; we'd never expected a magic cure (though we still wished for one). But the prospect of seeing those results on a PowerPoint presentation, with my little sister identified as patient six, scared the hell out of even my mother the superhero.

The presenter from the sponsor company arrived the day before the session and was shocked to learn that parents of two of the six trial patients were there.

"He said he didn't think parents would travel that far," Mom said to me after arriving home several days later, still in disbelief.

"What did you say?"

"I said, 'Come on. I'll go to the ends of the earth for this child. I did the trial, isn't that proof enough?'"

The presenter didn't understand the first thing about being the parent of a dying child, but he was considerate enough to share the data with my mom and the other parent who had traveled to Germany, and he invited them to breakfast before the public unveiling. *There was nothing shocking,* Mom said in a quick email to me after their conversation. *He said they can show the treatment has promise. Unfortunately that's because of the death of one of the children.*

The presenter announced the results to a crowd of people that afternoon, along with the PowerPoint slides Mom had dreaded. Though I was half a world away, I could picture my mother under the banquet hall's bright lights, scribbling notes. In my mind she looked friendly and approachable at first glance, but underneath her pretty smile and Southern charm she was tough as nails. She had a dying child, and she wasn't in the mood to take crap from anyone—including Batten disease and a biopharmaceutical company.

After the presentation in Germany, the study sponsor issued a news release about the trial. I was at work and my schedule was jam-packed, but when the news alert popped into my email, I shut down the project I'd been slogging through and closed my office door. Back at my desk, I ran my hands through my hair and took a deep breath. Though we had the inside track and Mom had already shared what she'd heard firsthand, somehow the formal release made it real. I needed a moment.

The official word was that high doses of stem cells were tolerated well and that the patients' conditions following transplantation "appeared consistent with the normal course of the disease." Because the second patient in the trial had died, they also knew that the stem cells she'd received had "engrafted and survived." At the end of the day, they'd gotten what they needed. The stem cells and the surgery to transplant them were safe.

I get it, I thought, closing my eyes. *We knew this was a safety trial—nothing more. We weren't sold on hope.* And yet nothing could have prepared me for a news release—a tool I used at work every day—that turned my living, breathing sister into a number, and a dying one to boot.

My eyes still closed, I remembered the cold night John and I arrived in Portland for Taylor's surgery. I remembered Mom and Dad pulling us into our hotel suite's kitchenette to tell us the news that the trial's other girl—there had been two girls and four boys—had passed away. I remembered how *healthy* my sister seemed on the surface in those days—obviously going blind, yes, but not terminally ill. I remembered getting that roller coaster feeling and not knowing at first if I was more scared of the stem cell treatment or my sister's surgery getting cancelled.

Signing on to the trial was one of the most frightening times of my life, Mom's last email from Germany said. *I have no regrets. I don't think it is the answer at this time, but I believe it has helped in some ways and given us important time.*

Time.

There was never enough time.

WHILE SHE WAS in Germany trying to save Taylor's life, my mother missed my sister's fifth grade graduation. I met Dad at The Fletcher School for the ceremony and clapped for my sister in the front row like a proud parent. Her teachers recognized her for her "inspirational attitude" and her "amazing accomplishment of learning braille."

Tears sprang to my eyes as Taylor made her way carefully up the stage steps with the help of a friend to receive her fifth grade certificate. Really—how many parents cry at these things?

Taylor would be eleven years old in August.

I'd always liked the number eleven. I wore the number eleven throughout my soccer career. I tacked it onto my name in email addresses and online usernames.

But eleven wasn't good enough. Taylor hadn't had her fill.

Chapter 10

I WASN'T SUPPOSED to be a runner.

The morning of my fourth day in the world, my mom saw what she thought might be a seizure, and it frightened her. She was twenty-four and new to parenting but intuitive enough to know something was wrong with her baby. I'd had jaundice, so fortunately we were still at the hospital. The next morning, the pediatrician told my parents they'd also observed seizure activity while I was in the nursery. I was moved to the intensive care unit for observation.

Brain imaging tests showed I'd suffered an intraventricular hemorrhage. Blood was leaking into the fluid-filled areas, called ventricles, causing pressure around my brain. Tiny blood clots had formed, blocking the normal flow of cerebrospinal fluid. The fluid had built up and caused hydrocephalus. My five-day-old brain was under abnormal pressure, which could lead to serious damage.

Before the end of my first week of life I'd had surgery: a pediatric neurosurgeon put in a shunt to drain the superfluous spinal fluid from my brain into my abdomen.

Somewhere in the midst of it all, Mom and Dad were told I might experience developmental delays and difficulties with movement as I grew up. I'd be shunt-dependent, and as I got older, I'd potentially need more surgeries in order to revise or replace the shunt. All of this put me at risk for cognitive deficits and physical handicaps. My parents were prepped for a long and difficult road with their first child—and my doctors weren't sure I'd ever walk problem-free, let alone run.

Three months later, I developed a shunt infection. The shunt had to be removed, and yet my doctors thought I'd likely still need a shunt to survive long-term. So they decided to treat the infection and put in a new shunt. Then, a wrinkle came. The shunt infection had caused a serious condition called ventriculitis—which by itself had a high mortality rate.

But when they removed the original shunt, my doctors discovered my body had cleared the hemorrhage on its own, and my brain was draining spinal fluid normally, independent of the shunt. With the infected shunt gone and my tiny body on a healthy dose of antibiotics, the ventriculitis went away, too.

They still don't know how that happened. But all I have left of the shunt—and the hemorrhage that could have killed or maimed me for life—are two tiny scars on my scalp and my belly.

I used to think everything happens for a reason. I liked the idea that God had some grand plan for me, that I'd been lucky because I was meant to do something great. Then when I was twenty-four, still searching for my place in the world, I learned my little sister was born with a tragic, fatal disease with no known cure.

I don't believe everything happens for a reason anymore.

In the early days following Taylor's diagnosis, I'd questioned God's choices: *Why us? Why her? Why our family?* It took me a while to realize I was asking the wrong questions. I wasn't helping anyone, least of all Taylor, by doubting genetics we couldn't change. I didn't really start fighting until I figured that out. For the first time, I understood the real question wasn't "Why her?" or "Why us?" but "What's next?" We can't always choose what happens to us in life, I'd learned. But we can choose how we act on it.

I WAS PONDERING this during a shower so hot the steam almost made me dizzy. It was Fourth of July weekend, and we'd driven to my Uncle David and Aunt Holly's house on Smith Mountain Lake in Virginia. I'd snuck out the front door for a short run while my family slept. The whole neighborhood had seemed to glisten with dew in the early morning light.

I rinsed the conditioner from my hair, the hot water running down my body in streams, when I felt it: a hard, smooth lump, about the size of a gumdrop, on the back of my neck. I felt a flutter in my chest.

"Take a look," I said to Uncle David minutes later, after I'd thrown on clothes and hurried downstairs. I turned my back to him and pointed to my neck, my hair still dripping wet. My uncle was perched on a barstool in the kitchen, wearing basketball shorts and a workout tee, devouring N.C. State athletics recruiting updates on his laptop. He'd turned forty the previous year but still looked thirty or even twenty-five—too young to be a neurosurgeon.

David touched the offending lump. He immediately looked concerned—not "Call 9-1-1 right now" concerned, but definitely "Have you had this examined?" concerned.

"That's your lymph node." He moved his fingers to the other side of my spine. "How long have you had this?"

"I don't know."

He rubbed his chin. "Well, it's probably nothing. Lymph nodes can swell for a lot of reasons. But you should get it checked out."

And that's how I ended up in a general surgeon's office barely two weeks later. By then, I'd made myself half crazy researching swollen lymph nodes on the Internet. Everything I'd read said they were usually caused by treatable infections, not cancer. But after my family's run of bad luck, a simple infection almost sounded too good to be true. When the surgeon examined me and recommended a biopsy, I wasn't surprised, but I also didn't feel any better. At the outpatient surgery center on an August morning the week before Taylor's eleventh birthday, I thought about telling the staff not to call me with the results unless they were good.

All I wanted was a break. I didn't think I could take Batten disease and cancer, too.

The phone call came on the fifth day after the biopsy. I was in a meeting and missed it; when I called back and asked to speak with my surgeon's nurse, the receptionist put me on hold. I half lay, half sat at my desk at work, straightening a paper clip with one hand and drawing lines in the dust on my computer monitor with the other. When the nurse finally came on the line, I jumped at the sound of her voice.

"Hello, are you still there?"

I'd forgotten I was holding the phone. I wondered how long she'd been waiting.

"Yes, I'm still here." My voice didn't sound right. I paused, expecting her to ask when I could come in to discuss the results in person.

"I have good news. The node was benign."

"I'm sorry—can you say that again?"

"You're okay. We'll mail a copy of your results, but you don't need to worry."

I thanked the nurse, my voice barely a whisper. Then, snapping back to reality, I heard myself asking mundane questions, such as "When can

I start running again?" and "Is it okay if I play soccer next week?" and "Can I take normal showers, or do I have to cover the sutures?" And the ghost of cancer drifted out of my life before we ever really got to know each other—just like that.

I was relieved; I know that much. But I'd spent so much time imagining the worst that I didn't know how to handle the good news.

The truth, as I began to realize on my drive home from the office that afternoon, was that I'd always taken my own health for granted, despite my rough start in the world. I'd always assumed that tomorrow, I'd still be able to run and see and talk.

My brief cancer scare reminded me that I couldn't take a single day for granted. But even if that call had been different—if the nurse had asked me to come in to discuss the results in person—I'd have had options, at least. I'd have had experts with the ability to give me the best shot decades of research could buy: maybe not a cure, but access to treatments that had kept a lot of people alive and well for a long time.

The cold reality, I knew, was that my sister didn't have that luxury.

MY MOTHER WAS doing her best to give Taylor a chance at a full life. I was doing everything I thought I had the capacity to do, and yet I wanted to be more like my mom. There were days I felt I wasn't angry or focused or inspired enough.

I called Mom one night to check in.

"I found a flight to St. Louis," she said right away. Her voice had a no-nonsense edge to it, though underneath the armor I heard fatigue.

The Batten Association's annual conference was being held in St. Louis.

"I thought we decided to take a break again this year," I replied.

"Well, I'm going. My flight leaves in the morning."

A beat passed.

"What made you change your mind?"

"I got a call from Doug Smith. Do you remember the Smiths?"

Mom and Dad had first met Doug and his wife Cindy at the lysosomal disease symposium in 2006. They'd traveled all the way to Orlando from Winnipeg, Canada, searching for answers for their son Brandon, who, like Taylor, had infantile Batten disease.

"I do," I answered, seeing Brandon's picture in my mind. He had short brown hair, porcelain skin, and delicate features that hinted at the happy, smiling, laughing boy he'd once been.

"Doug was sorry we didn't make last year's conference," Mom continued. "He said, 'The work of Taylor's Tale helped give hope to children like my son.' He told me it didn't feel whole without us—that we needed to be there."

And that's how my mother ended up going back on her promise to give herself a rest, instead awarding research grants to Sandy Hofmann and two other investigators at the National Institutes of Health and Washington University in St. Louis—in person. We were funding work at a level that represented a big leap of faith for our fledgling charity, still less than a year removed from filing the paperwork to establish our non-profit status. But Taylor's Tale had helped inspire a movement among other families battling my sister's form of the disease, historically the least well-funded of the major forms of Batten disease; for the first time in anyone's memory, and maybe the first time ever, four research projects for infantile Batten disease received funding at the Batten Association conference.

John and I picked my mother up from the airport late on a Sunday afternoon so Dad could stay home with Taylor. Smells of summer—grass clippings and grilled meat and sunscreen—filled the air. Even as we approached the airport, the streets were quiet. The world was at play. But then we walked inside baggage claim and found Mom standing by the door with her rolling suitcase and computer bag, checking emails on her phone, and I remembered the world that took it easy on a summer day wasn't the world my mother lived in.

"How are you?" I asked, hugging her.

"These conferences haven't grown on me any since Rochester." Her makeup was perfect, but her eyes looked even more tired than usual.

"But you're glad you went?"

"Doug was right," she said with conviction. "This fight needs us."

OF MY PARENTS, I'd been closer to my father for as long as I could remember. Mom was an advocate years before she had a daughter with a fatal disease; throughout my childhood and early teenage years, she pulled long nights at community non-profit board meetings and events on top of her day job as a piano teacher. Dad, Stephen, and I used to eat grilled cheese sandwiches for dinner, then skip down the aisles at the grocery store getting the items on Mom's list plus our special picks. Often we'd end the night at the Baskin Robbins in the mall for ice cream cones—mint chocolate chip for me, and chocolate chip cookie dough for them. The mall had a fountain with benches, and we'd take our cones and throw pennies into the spray until Dad's pockets were empty. My father cheered at all of my soccer games; on weekends we shared the sports page and the comics; he taught me to fish and helped me count the stars at father-daughter camp.

Now that I was an adult, things had changed. I was with my mother far more often. It had started with planning my wedding. We'd talked every day—about venues, caterers, florists, musicians, and bridesmaids' dresses—everything mothers and daughters talk about when the daughter is engaged.

I'd barely had time to unpack after the honeymoon when we got the diagnosis. Mom and I still talked daily after that, but our conversations weren't so happy anymore. Usually we talked about Taylor's Tale; sometimes I felt like we were more colleagues than relatives. Mom was always thinking about how to beat Batten disease, and I was her sounding board. On the other hand, Dad and I didn't talk as much anymore after we got the news, partly because I'd grown up and stayed busy but mostly, I think, because he was sad. Unlike my mother, who tends to go at life's problems like a wolverine, my father is like an ostrich that sticks its head in the sand at any sign of danger.

We celebrated Taylor's eleventh birthday on a Wednesday night. John and I parked and snuck into my parents' open garage to hide her large gift—an electric keyboard for a music lover who "saw" with her fingers—and stow the ice cream cake we'd brought in the second freezer. The garage lights were dimmed, and we each jumped a foot in the air when we heard a clatter in the other bay.

"Dad?" I reached behind the old refrigerator and flicked on the overhead light. My father was sitting on one of his well-worn Masters golf chairs surrounded by ancient shoeboxes next to the sagging shelves, sorting through stacks of photos by the glow of a flashlight.

"Oh, hey there." He glanced up and managed a smile. He looked as though he was noticing us for the first time.

"I'm going to see if your mom needs anything," John said quickly, as if sensing that we might need a moment. "See you inside."

I dropped my purse on a pile of dusty gym bags and walked across the garage. When I put my hand on Dad's shoulder, he looked up at me. The light shone directly on his face; the crow's feet edging his green eyes looked more pronounced than ever, and his hair was grayer than I remembered. How quickly can you age? My father had always won the "guess your age" contests at the state fair because he looked so young. After a couple of times, Mom made a rule that we couldn't play that game until the end of the night, because everyone had to take a turn carrying the enormous stuffed animal prize.

"Are you okay?" My voice pierced the silence.

"Do you remember going to Hornets games?"

For years my Grandma Margaret and Granddaddy Parks had had season tickets for the Charlotte Hornets NBA team, and Dad and I had gone to almost every home game.

"I do. Those teams had some good players. And they sold out every game. That place was loud." I noticed then that he was holding a picture of us on the concourse at the old coliseum, demolished a few years after the original Hornets left town for New Orleans my sophomore year of college. A much younger version of my dad, a guy with the same smile but smooth skin and dark brown—not gray—hair, had his arm around me. My hair, long and stringy and platinum blonde, was streaming out from a too-big Hornets cap. I wore a purple and teal Hornets t-shirt and the black stirrup pants I favored in elementary school, and I had a huge grin on my face. I realized that I looked like a blonder version of my sister. I must have been about eleven in the photo. *He's thinking about Taylor,* I said to myself. *It's her birthday and time's moving too quickly and he's thinking of all they won't share.*

We stayed there for a minute in the stillness, neither of us ready to climb the stairs and join the celebratory commotion. I wished we could stay down in that garage and talk basketball—maybe even head out to the driveway after the heavy August air had dissipated and play a game of H-O-R-S-E. But Dad put the photos back in the box and stood up, and we hugged and started for the door. His eyes were red-rimmed and moist, but he didn't cry. I went first, soundless, taking my time, hoping the night would last forever, as if by not blowing out her candles my sister could keep the monster away.

THE WEEKEND AFTER the birthday party, Dad and Stephen headed to Raleigh with two cars loaded up, signaling the beginning of my brother's senior year of college.

I'd promised to keep Mom and Taylor company in my father's absence. Taylor wanted a new backpack for middle school, so we went to the mall. My mother and I described, in minute detail, the colors and patterns of each and every girls' backpack at a luggage specialty shop.

"This one has orange polka dots," I said, holding up a daypack with wheels.

Taylor shook her head. "I want pink."

"What about this one?" Mom asked from across the aisle. She held out a pink and green plaid backpack and let Taylor feel the pattern's raised texture.

My sister shook her head so hard I thought she might fall into the shelving unit. "All pink."

That was that. Mom summoned a salesperson, who helped us find an all-pink backpack with padding for Taylor's new laptop outfitted with special software for the blind. The cashier offered to give us a large plastic bag, but my sister wanted to wear her new pack to the car.

That afternoon, we headed to the pool, where we sat side by side on a towel spread out by the water's edge. We shared a bag of kettle corn and sipped five-calorie Crystal Light as the August sun dipped behind the trees, signaling the unofficial end of summer.

I inspected my chipped toenail polish in the cool, clear water and turned to my sister. "What if I treat you to a pedicure for the first day of school?"

But Taylor had bigger things on her mind.

"When do I get to drive?"

Mom and I exchanged glances over Taylor's head.

"Not for a couple of years. What made you think of that?"

"When I get my license, I want a pink convertible, like Sharpay from *High School Musical.*"

Mom didn't hesitate. "Taylor, honey, if you get your driver's license, you will have your pink convertible, by God—even if it has to be custom-painted."

SEVERAL WEEKS INTO the school year, Taylor got her first progress report. By then she was only taking two classes—reading comprehension and social studies—in addition to the one-on-one work she did with her vision teacher, Jill Fowler. She'd gotten a ninety-eight average in both subjects.

"You're awesome, Taylor," I said when Dad showed me the report. "I'm so proud of you." I wrapped my arms around her in a bear hug. She didn't hug me back; instead she stood there, still as a statue.

"What's wrong?" I pulled away and searched her face.

"Ninety-eight isn't very good."

"Ninety-eight is great. It's an A."

"But Miss Jill says one hundred is perfect."

What does "perfect" mean? Nobody's perfect. I'd gotten high test scores all my life, but I couldn't follow a recipe and still got lost in my hometown. I'd escaped getting Batten disease, but I had rickety joints and migraine headaches.

Anyone unhappy with a ninety-eight is an overachiever, I thought. But what was so wrong with that? After all, Taylor had taught me there's no such thing as over-achieving. If we aren't willing to test the limits of our minds and bodies—if we're afraid to stretch our belief of what's possible—what do we have?

"Listen, T," I said, pulling her close again. "Ninety-eight is awesome. But if you're going for a hundred, you'll do it. I know you will."

IN OCTOBER, JOHN and I flew to the red rock canyons of Utah and the soaring vistas of the Grand Canyon's North Rim for a much-needed vacation—our first together since our honeymoon.

At home, life was a blur of work and meetings and eternal to-do lists. I'd started a one-year term as president of Taylor's Tale at the beginning of August, and the administrative tasks of running a public charity, even a small one, zapped me more than building awareness—a huge task but one I felt better equipped to handle. I smiled at Taylor's Tale events, but

I gritted my teeth as I put in long hours on my computer for our charity each night after leaving my day job. I found that as much passion as I had for telling my sister's story to the world, I didn't like managing volunteers, planning and running board meetings, or making sure we filed our taxes on time. Worst of all, I was never satisfied with my efforts. I worried that if I waited one too many days to answer an email or didn't craft the perfect blog post, I'd be hurting my sister's chance at survival. Life moved so quickly and weighed so heavily on me, I rarely noticed the rise and fall of the sun.

But out west, tucked into remote canyons far from cell phone towers and computers and boardrooms, I found I could breathe. I didn't exactly slow down—we hiked over eighty miles in seven days—but I was present. I saw the ribbons of color in walls plunging toward canyon floors and twisted, ancient branches, stark against a clear blue sky.

The day we drove from Utah to Arizona, I got up early and ran alone alongside a canyon filled with pillars of stone. Like giant drip castles frozen in time, they caught the morning sunlight on smooth rock faces the color of fire and sand. I held on to the images in my brain. The blood coursed through my body, and the cold air filled my lungs. A raven called from far below. And I started remembering. Memories of making snow angels with my sister in a pile of leaves. Floating on our backs in the shallow end of the pool, our eyes squeezed shut to the unforgiving summer sun. Swinging as high as we could, till our feet touched heaven.

"Taylor won't get to see anything like this," I said to my husband on our last night. We were shivering in front of the huge stone fireplace on the terrace of our lodge overlooking the Grand Canyon. Above us were more stars than I'd ever seen in my lifetime, like they'd been spattered across a black canvas from a can of iridescent white paint. It was the first time I'd ever seen the Milky Way.

"I never want to leave this place," I whispered, burrowing into John's heavy coat as the fire winked out. But even as I said the words, I knew I didn't mean them. I felt renewed and alive, and I couldn't wait to start fighting again.

WHEN JOHN AND I returned home, autumn had arrived in Charlotte, and with the change of seasons I could sense a change in Taylor, too.

Halloween had always been Taylor's favorite holiday, which made sense for a girl who loved playing dress-up. This year she'd asked to be a queen bee, and with Mom's help she'd designed her own costume. She came bounding awkwardly down the steps right as John and I walked through the front door. My sister looked memorable in her yellow and black-striped tights, black leotard, glittery wings, fuzzy antennae, and gold Mardi Gras beads.

I made a mental note not to take too many pictures, afraid I'd miss the moment if I hid behind my camera all night.

"Is it time to trick-or-treat yet?" she asked, stumbling a bit on the words—a new symptom.

I twisted to look behind me at the rain pelting the street outside. "Just about," I said.

"There should be a break soon," John told us, showing me the Doppler radar map on his phone.

Sure enough, the rain granted us a thirty-minute break not long after we arrived. Dad, John, and I took Taylor door-to-door while my mother stayed behind to distribute candy. At most of the houses, I hung back with Dad while John held my sister's arm and helped her navigate winding walkways, steep steps, and tricky landscaping. Watching her strain to find her way to the neighbors' front doors and take the candy they offered, I thought about how, on the eve of the first Halloween after the diagnosis, I'd worried if my sister's poor night vision would prevent her from trick-or-treating. But her vision now was gone, and I didn't worry about it anymore. Instead, I wondered how much longer she'd be able to walk the neighborhood streets and ring doorbells before Batten disease stole her legs from her, too.

I knew that soon, it would be three years since our first fundraiser. And while science had come a long way since we founded Taylor's Tale, we were still running from Batten disease. Portland and the stem cells hadn't saved my sister, and we didn't have anything better waiting in the wings.

We reached my parents' driveway just as a light rain began to fall. The wind picked up, scattering the leaves that had fallen that day. I shuddered, but I'm not sure if it was from the cold.

THE NEXT DAY, Brandon Smith from Winnipeg died in his parents' arms. He was eight years old. When Mom called me, I cried, swallowed up by sadness and anger and fear and incomprehension.

In the weeks that followed, Brandon's mother, Cindy, contacted my mother and talked to her about a donation. They'd done some fundraising over the past several years, and memorial gifts had come in since Brandon's passing.

"The Smiths are donating the funds to Taylor's Tale," Mom told me.

"That's wonderful," I answered.

She didn't say anything for a moment, then, "They're sending a check for $20,000."

I couldn't speak. I understood then, maybe better than ever, that we'd been given an amazing opportunity to make a difference, and that families sitting where we sat trusted us to lead them out of the darkness.

That night, I ran like I'd never run before. I ran until my legs ached and my chest burned, and when I collapsed on the sofa later, I didn't care that I was sticky with sweat.

IT WAS FREEZING the morning of the Thunder Road Half Marathon, and John and I drove uptown alone. I hated the waiting; I just wanted to run.

Soon after sunrise, I got my wish.

I coasted on endorphins for the first several miles. Then, at mile five, my body fought back. I felt a fire raging in the balls of my feet and tightness clenching in my calves. By mile eight, spectators were encouraging me to grind it out. I wished I hadn't played hurt so many times in my soccer career. I wished I'd spent more of the past few months training and less time on my laptop.

By mile twelve, my chest hurt, and my breath was shallow. I tried to think about the rest of the race as four laps around a track. After two "laps," I started searching in vain for the finish line.

I could see the mile thirteen marker in the distance when I first seriously considered walking. At that moment, a woman watching from the sidewalk called to me, gesturing ahead.

"Once you turn that corner, you'll be able to see the finish line."

My legs and my lungs hurt so badly, it didn't seem possible for me to run the rest of the way. Then, I remembered what Mary-Kate had told me at the finish line of the Thunder Road 5K a year earlier.

Your sister never wanted to walk. Even when she fell and scraped her knees. She just pulled herself up and started running again.

For me, right then, that close to the end, walking felt like quitting. It felt like giving up. Deep down I knew it was crazy, but I viewed giving up on running as equal to giving up on Taylor—much the way I viewed taking a night off from Taylor's Tale when I could be answering emails from donors or writing my blog.

I turned the corner, and I saw the finish line—just like the woman on the sidewalk had promised. Though my body begged me to stop, I sprinted the last one-tenth of a mile to the finish.

I was so exhausted that I almost didn't recognize John as he put an arm around me. Dizzy with fatigue, I reached up to wipe sweat from my face, only to find I'd been crying. When had that happened?

I realized I'd just run my first half marathon. I hadn't finished with a great time, yet I'd become a long-distance runner. I'd always been a sprinter first. But similar to our fight against Batten disease, I'd come to understand the value of a long-term plan. I'd learned how to push my body past the limits of what I'd previously believed it could achieve.

And yet, my sister's body was failing her.

Shoulders slumped, I took my medal and walked toward the car.

Chapter 11

LOOKING BACK, I think the winter that followed that race may have been my lowest point since the diagnosis. The trees that bordered my favorite running route had been stripped of their leaves, resembling lonely, twisted scarecrows in the gray cold. Like the trees, we'd been stripped bare, used up. Taylor's Tale had lost its shiny newness, and my sister's own light was fading. More and more, I caught myself staring at photos of her in my home office late at night, the cursor impatiently blinking on a blank meeting agenda or blog post or press release or whatever I needed to be doing. In all of the photos, Taylor had long blonde hair and looked at the camera.

For me, our fight against Batten disease had developed into a great paradox: running a charity was hard, but losing Taylor would be harder—and I knew in my heart that if we quit, there would be no one waiting in the wings to continue the fight for us. I understood that if we wanted to save my sister, we'd have to lead the charge.

So I kept going. Meanwhile, my twenty-something peers spent their free time with friends and focused on their careers and went to grad school and had babies. When I felt angry or sad, I ran, my lungs burning from the cold.

In mid-January, Daniel Kerner turned ten years old. Each of the previous four years, he'd celebrated by tucking into an adaptive bi-ski and skiing down California's Mammoth Mountain. But this year, Daniel's condition had deteriorated enough that the Kerners kept him home, instead marking the day with cake and ice cream in a warm kitchen. I thought about driving to the North Carolina mountains and making a run for Daniel, but I decided I had too much to do.

I felt a kind of sadness that I couldn't explain. Maybe it was accepting that the Portland trial hadn't saved Taylor. Maybe it was the realization that I'd given up so much of my own life—years I couldn't get back—and yet I could still lose what mattered most to me when it was all over.

I GOT A boost the last day of February, when piano teachers and students in my mother's hometown put on a piano play-a-thon in Taylor's honor. My parents and Taylor piled into my Explorer with us for the three-hour drive to Raleigh, where Stephen met us for the afternoon.

My grandmother's best friend Polly co-hosted the event, and I'd grown up around many of her relatives and friends who came to hear the students play. The recital halls were awash in purple—purple balloons, purple confetti, purple plates and cups and napkins—for Taylor's Tale. A lot of the kids—even some of the boys—wore purple. I felt as if we'd been wrapped in an indestructible blanket of love and hope, at least temporarily. So many things felt like old times: the faces of people we'd joined for progressive dinners at Christmastime mixed in with kind strangers whose kids played their hearts out for my sister. Grandma Kathryn and Papa Jerry had driven up from the retirement home an hour away in Greensboro, and my grandmother beamed when Taylor laughed and clapped in time to the music. I tried not to focus on my grandmother's posture, droopy from the Lewy body dementia, or my sister's blindness.

Sometime that afternoon—I don't know when—one of the teenage students had learned that my sister loved the song "You Belong With Me" by Taylor Swift. He and a friend found me in the back of the room by the information table after he played his planned pieces.

"Would it be alright if we played a Taylor Swift song for your sister?"

I looked up from the brochures I'd been straightening and gazed up at them. The one who'd spoken had shaggy, dark hair that fell into his eyes. And his friend was so tall. He was holding a cello.

"Umm . . ." I felt tears pricking the backs of my eyes. I tried to guess the age difference between these guys and my sister. I'd have expected high school kids to be playing video games or basketball or hanging out at the mall on a Sunday afternoon.

"That would make Taylor so happy," I said, finding my voice again. "Thank you."

Throughout the song—which the teenagers played beautifully—I watched Taylor's face. Though she'd laughed and clapped all day, she was silent for those four minutes. She didn't know to look toward the stage, so others might have thought she'd zoned out. But I knew that when Taylor got quiet, she was listening, focusing all of her energy and attention and the senses she still had on the thing that mattered most in that moment. She cocked her head as she concentrated on the music—a habit she'd formed after she lost all but her peripheral vision, forcing her to view the world through the corners of her eyes.

It was as if someone had switched on a light inside of her. She lived in darkness. But she saw everything.

IN MIDDLE SCHOOL, I hadn't exactly been at the top of the social food chain. I read thick paperbacks and wrote science fiction stories and liked sports, none of which granted me access to the popular table in the school cafeteria. I didn't have boyfriends—I had friends who were boys. We played pickup basketball and argued over who should bat cleanup for the Atlanta Braves. Nonetheless, I wanted to fit in.

I hated dresses, but I got a skirt and matching blouse for the eighth grade social and went with three also dateless girlfriends. The floor of the school's lobby had been buffed to a high sheen, and the main hallways were closed off. Celine Dion and R. Kelly and other mid-nineties icons warbled from compact speakers. Black and orange confetti lit up long tables stacked high with store-bought brownies and tropical punch. My friends and I stood near the punch bowl and refilled our cups whenever we thought we'd been standing for too long. One of the girls dared me to talk to my crush—a forward on the boys' soccer team—but instead I watched him flirt with two cheerleaders from a safe distance.

Taylor had no such insecurities. She went to her first middle school dance decked out in a sparkly pink and purple top adorned with dream catchers over a denim skirt, chocolate tights, and trendy UGG boots. The Fletcher School staff had asked me to come to the dance and watch out for her; the sixth graders had strictly forbidden parents from the school grounds during the dance, but, as an older sister, I was allowed.

I'd never worried that my sister's classmates would be cruel to her. I'd only worried that they would be human—that they would get caught up in their own lives, and that Taylor, blind and struggling to string together cohesive thoughts and long sentences as her speech processing skills declined, would simply miss the wave.

But as I stood against the wall in the darkened school cafeteria, neon deejay lights painting the air and the front of my shirt, I thought about Taylor's Girls on the Run experience and pizza outings and sleepovers, and I thanked God for the kids who'd illuminated my sister's world with small acts of great love.

Having never attended a dance with a date until my junior prom when I was seventeen, I got to bear witness for the first time, thanks to my little sister, the best parts of crushing on a boy pre-high school. I'd expected to twirl Taylor around the cafeteria floor just like our dance parties at home, but instead she spent most of the night on the arm of her crush, Scott Wallace. The rest of the boys did their best to avoid the opposite sex; instead of brushing up on their dance moves, they stood around by the pretzels and plates of chocolate chip cookies, talking about soccer team tryouts and pizza toppings and, when they thought no one was listening, which girls looked the prettiest.

Scott was friendly with all of those guys, but he never left Taylor. He took her hands and led her around the room in an awkward, pre-teen version of the waltz. Whenever her girlfriends called her name and drew her into their circle of laughter and bouncing, he'd hand her off to my sister's friend, Charlotte, and dash off just long enough to grab a handful of pretzel sticks or a soda, which he'd offer to Taylor. Then, he'd lead her back to the rear of the cafeteria—where they had less chance of falling or bumping into their classmates—and twirl her around again.

Taylor couldn't see and Scott had no rhythm, but I thought it was one of the most beautiful things I'd ever witnessed.

RUNNING SUSTAINED ME through the winter season, and though I hadn't been thinking past Thunder Road, I found I couldn't wait to race again. So in April, I ran a ten-mile race for Taylor on the streets of Chapel Hill and the campus of my alma mater, the University of North Carolina. The chilly, dew-kissed air danced on my skin as hot pink and white azaleas, blooming dogwoods, and buildings older than the Constitution whizzed by.

I felt better prepared for the ten-mile distance than for the half marathon I'd run at Thunder Road four months earlier; halfway through the course, my body coasted and my mind wandered. I remembered the day I'd graduated from college on the campus where I was now running. My sister was small, and her powder blue dress covered with tiny blue flowers came nearly to the ground, so that her toes just barely peeked out from her strappy white sandals. I'd pulled her close in the crowd outside the stadium after the ceremony. In my daydream, I watched as she took my hand and I placed my too-large cap on her head. The image faded just as she smiled, her bright eyes lighting up the world.

Back then, I couldn't have known my sister was unlikely to ever wear a cap and gown of her own. I couldn't have known she'd been set up to lose everything. As I snapped back to the present, running through a tunnel and into the sun-filled football stadium with the terrible knowledge of all that Batten disease had stolen from Taylor, I was furious. I didn't think about any of the good Taylor still had. Instead, I only saw the bad, angry and red in my vision field. I pumped my arms and legs as if I was punching the monster with every stride. I sprinted around the track, passing a bunch of people who'd led me the whole race. I lunged across the finish line like I was being chased by demons.

I didn't come close to winning the race. But I'd shaved three minutes per mile off my December half marathon pace, and I didn't even feel like I was going to throw up afterward. I hadn't gotten a great time, but I didn't care. For that day at least, I'd achieved my running goal.

I knew I had less room for error where Batten disease was concerned, though. I didn't want to finish in the middle of the pack. And as I collapsed next to John in the stadium bleachers, the sun glinting off the race medal around my neck, I understood my deep winter funk. I'd seen and felt a change in Taylor since the previous year, and I was terrified that we were in danger of running out of time. I'd become obsessed with winning the race that really mattered. Because I knew that if we lost, or if we didn't finish quickly enough, one day I'd lie awake in bed at night, wishing I could hold my little sister close again.

DANIEL PASSED AWAY the day after I crossed the finish line in Chapel Hill.

I slumped over my laptop late that night, mocked by another wretched blinking cursor and blank page, my bags from the weekend still not unpacked and dirty laundry in a pile in the floor. In the space between moonset and dawn, I wrote a letter.

Dear Daniel,

There must be lots of mountains to ski down in heaven. Are they as beautiful as Mammoth Mountain? As you're racing down the slopes, feel the wind in your hair and the sun on your face, but also the presence of your family and friends. They love you so much, and they will always be by your side.

You and my little sister, Taylor, have so much in common! Just like you wouldn't let Batten disease stop you from going to the ocean and skiing, Taylor hasn't let Batten disease stop her from going to school with her friends or singing and dancing.

I am afraid of Batten disease, but Taylor helps me stay strong, just like you help your mommy and daddy stay strong. It's easy to want to fight for fighters like you and Taylor. You are my heroes. I write lots of stories about Taylor, and I even wrote a story about you when you turned ten years old in January.

I am so sorry we weren't able to find a cure for Batten disease in time to save you, Daniel. Everyone already misses you here, but you are with God now, and I know He will keep you safe. Your life inspired so many people, and I know it will help give me the strength I need to keep fighting for Taylor and all of the other children with Batten disease.

Your mommy told me that after your surgery, she felt like she was seeing the brilliant sunlight of hope for the first time. Even though your body has left us now, Daniel, your spirit still burns brightly. I'm not surprised that someone who loves adventures as much as you do would bring so much hope to so many people. Your life was a miracle. And one day, because of the gifts you gave us, I will find mine.

I didn't feel hopeful, though. I floated downstairs like a ghost, my bare feet hardly skimming the carpeted stairs, and slid into bed without washing my face. That night, I had a dream.

Taylor and I were on a carousel. My sister was healthy, with golden skin and hair and a toothy smile that lit up her young face. She perched atop a handsome white stallion, its hand-carved saddle and bridle painted in dazzling colors that glistened in the summer sun and the carousel's gilded mirrors. The ride began to move, the notes of its Wurlitzer organ dancing on the breeze. It spun faster and faster. Taylor's tiny fingers tightened around the bridle. She tossed her head back, laughing. But no sound came from her. And when the carousel came to a stop, I was standing alone, and the great stallion's bridle hung limply in the pale light of dusk.

Chapter 12

MAY BROUGHT SHOWERS to our corner of the world, and kindness bloomed like my mother's hydrangeas and dogwoods and the cherry blossom trees in the park where Taylor and I used to feed the ducks. My outlook started to brighten with the change in seasons.

"The Fletcher kids had two fundraisers for Taylor's Tale," Mom said on the phone one afternoon as I drove home from my office at the hospital.

"That's great. What did they do?" The traffic light glowed red. I rested my foot on the brake and watched middle school students play soccer in a field across the street.

"The kids ran the show. They got approval from the powers that be, and they organized and promoted both events. Friday, T's classmates wore pajamas to school in return for a one-dollar donation. The girls sold snacks during lunch, too."

The light turned green. "How did they do?"

"In the carpool line, T's friends handed me an envelope decorated with purple flowers and hearts. It was stuffed so full, they'd had to tape it shut." Mom paused.

"And?"

"There was almost five hundred dollars in that envelope."

I grinned and pictured my sister's girlfriends selling popcorn and juice boxes. "What about the other fundraiser?"

"The girls in the grade below your sister are wrapping up Girls on the Run," she said. "They had a bake sale in the lobby today."

I stopped at another light. "And?"

"You should have seen them, Laura. They decorated pink and purple posters with glitter and flowers and information about Batten disease and ran up to all of the parents and teachers to tell them about Taylor's Tale. They're younger than your sister and they don't really know her that well but they were all so excited to sell cookies and cupcakes for her. Would you believe they raised seven hundred and fifty dollars in an hour?"

Years later, I'm still moved by the kindness of my sister's classmates. They didn't look at my sister in a certain way. They didn't scream in her ear as if she was deaf, just because she was blind. They didn't tease her for running races with a guide. They didn't notice when she stumbled over her words. They never treated her like she was dying. I've often thought Taylor's friends, when they were young, were better at dealing with her illness than many adults.

Of course, from the outside, it's difficult to know what to say to someone facing a monster like Batten disease. I get that. I've never thought my friends had it easy.

I remember walking to the hospital parking deck with a friend one night after work a few weeks following the diagnosis. "You know," she said, resting her hand on my arm, "there *is* a silver lining in all of this."

"What's that?" I stopped looking for my car keys and searched her face in the parking deck's dim light.

"Getting through this—it's not going to be easy. But your friends will be here for you. And when you come out on the other side, you'll be a stronger person."

"Maybe so," I said, after a pause. "But I'd rather be an asshole if I knew that it meant my little sister wouldn't die." Part of what she said, of course, was true. Over the years many of my friends would stick with me through the worst of my sister's illness. But finding gain in my sister's loss felt like the ultimate betrayal. I didn't *want* anything from Batten disease. It just felt wrong, and I refused to go there.

I went to counseling for a while, first through a service for employees at the hospital and later at a private practice. My mother tried therapy, but she quit going after a few months. "I just don't like talking about it at predetermined times," she said. "It" being my sister's illness and its cataclysmic effect on our family. "I feel worse when I leave than when I walked in the door."

Actually, I didn't dread appointments with my therapists, though some days I'll admit the conversation felt forced. But I learned this: there didn't have to be any *reason* for Taylor to be sick. We could choose to make the best of what we'd been given. We could trust that God would give us the strength needed to fight the worst of what we had. But Batten disease had no silver lining.

I PLAYED ON a women's soccer team in the spring and fall, and the day after the bake sale at Fletcher, we had a late game. The sky was already black as ink as we stretched on the sidelines prior to the start of the match. As we were about to take the field, the floodlights winked out, leaving us in the dark. Somebody found a cell phone and called the league manager's office. The conversation drifted in a million directions while we waited for a league representative to arrive and restore the field lights. One of our defenders, Holly, mentioned she wanted to sell her three tickets to the musical *Wicked*.

"Three tickets?" I repeated. I knew Taylor would love the Broadway show about the witches of Oz. For years she'd collected *Wizard of Oz* snow globes, and she'd wanted to see the musical since hearing about it from our friend, Callie.

"Three tickets. They were eighty dollars apiece, but you can have them for sixty-five dollars each."

"My little sister is sick, and she'd give anything to go," I said, thinking how much she'd love the music even though her vision was long gone. "I'll buy them."

Holly's expression softened. "I remember hearing about your sister last season. I'm glad you can take her."

We had another game three nights later, so I showed up at the field with a check for one hundred ninety-five dollars. "Walk with me for a second," Holly said, when I knelt to slip the check in her bag. She stood up and led me away from the circle of women lacing up cleats and pulling socks over shin guards.

"Listen," she said, lowering her voice. "I don't need your check."

"What do you mean?"

"Someone on the team bought the tickets for you."

My heart fluttered. Automatically, I looked back over my shoulder at my teammates. They were all nice girls, but I wasn't particularly close to any of them. *There is good in the world,* I thought. *Even in a world that includes Batten disease.*

"Who?"

"I can't say." Holly threw an arm around me. "I hope your sister really likes *Wicked.*"

In every photo I have from the night of the musical, Taylor is beaming, her smile framed by soft, thick curls. For me, the most beautiful part of the performance had to be when Elphaba, the Wicked Witch of the West and the star of the show, rose high above the stage, crowned by an eerily beautiful blue light, her voice like an angel's. But I'll always remember how my little sister squeezed my hand and laughed out loud at the "baaaaahs" of Doctor Dillamond, the talking goat professor.

I still don't think that Batten disease has a silver lining. But I do believe this: those field lights went out for a reason.

THE PORTLAND STEM cell trial may not have saved my sister, but it had its own unexpected silver lining. For seven weeks during Taylor's surgery and recovery in 2008 and during each pre-op and return visit, my family had stayed in a Marriott Residence Inn at the foot of Oregon Health & Science University's Pill Hill. The trial sponsor had paid my family's expenses, but Mom and Dad were the ones who acquired the thousands of hotel rewards points, and by the summer of 2010, they had enough to take us all to the Virgin Islands for a four-day vacation during the Caribbean's low season.

"Request time off and pack your bags," Dad said when we met for coffee on a weekday afternoon in June. "We're going next month." What he didn't have to say was that we needed to hurry and go before my sister got any sicker.

I gazed at him and nodded slowly. He sensed my surprise—my father had never been a planner, yet here he was, orchestrating a major family vacation. "We can do it," he said. "Our points are good for a two-bedroom villa on St. Thomas. The only catch is that it's a timeshare property, and one morning your mom and I will have to go on a tour and pretend we're interested in buying into the place."

I smiled. "I wouldn't mind having a place in the Virgin Islands."

"Neither would I. But I'll settle for four days."

And that's how I ended up returning to St. Thomas—the island where John and I had honeymooned—only this time I came with my family in tow and with all of the scrapes and bruises that four years of fighting Batten disease had inflicted.

The newly built resort wasn't five-star quality, but it had sparkling pools and emerald green grass and a white-sand beach that sloped gently down to turquoise water. Wild iguanas roamed the resort grounds, feasting on dropped French fries and pineapple chunks and climbing on potted tropical plants. The days were warm and the nights were cool. After sunset, thousands of stars spattered the black sky that hung above the dark silhouettes of small islands like a painter's canvas.

Our first full day in the Caribbean, John and Stephen led Taylor down to the water's edge. Soft waves lapped against the shore, leaving foam like the head from a bottle of root beer. The ocean was shallow and calm, not like the angry waves of the Atlantic at the beaches back home. The boys took Taylor's wrists and led her toward the water. She dug the balls of her feet into the sand and tried to slip out of my brother's grasp, but she was smiling.

"Come on, T," John said. "This'll be fun." He pointed to the rainbow of coral scattered just beneath the water's surface. "Hey, Stephen," he said to my brother. "Let's lift her over that."

I followed them into the surf. The July sun was hot, but a soft breeze raised goose bumps on my wet skin. I went in up to my chest and leaned backward till my head touched the cool water. The water covered my ears and their voices and the sounds of the resort—a volleyball game in the pool, shouted orders at the grill—became muffled.

When I was little, my father used to tell me he could swim across the ocean. He would leave me standing by our beach chairs and sand buckets and dive into the mouth of a wave and disappear for a long time. Once I didn't think he was coming back, but then just as I went to tug on my mother's cover-up, he came walking up the beach, dripping wet and holding a sand dollar, which he gave to me. When I got a little older he'd take me out past the waves with him, and we'd float on our backs and give each other new names and imagine we'd been shipwrecked and were drifting to a magical new world where bad things never happened.

By the time I grew up, we'd stopped telling stories.

A sudden movement and a loud squeal jolted me back to the present. John had his arms around Taylor, and Stephen was tugging at his snorkel and mask.

"Was that a shark?" my brother asked.

Taylor squealed again.

"Yeah! I was telling T about this cute little sea bass," John said. "It was hanging out with us. Then this shark comes from out of nowhere and bites the damn thing in half."

Stephen and I whipped our heads around, suddenly on high alert.

"Where is it?" I said.

"It took off with its kill," John said.

"Should we be worried?" Stephen asked. The mask was still pinching his nose, and his voice sounded nasal.

"I don't think so. It was a little shark."

"Good answer."

"Come on, T," John said, taking my sister's hand again. "Let's go get a fruity drink and sit by the pool."

"Okay," Taylor said. She grabbed ahold of John's arm and let him lead her toward the shore. Stephen slid his mask down again and ducked underwater. I lingered, watching the rays of sunlight as they danced in the clear water and on the smooth white sand of the ocean floor.

Then, I saw the sea bass' body, torn in half and floating by the rocks. The shark was nowhere to be seen. But there was the poor fish, its life ripped away in the blink of an eye.

BETWEEN SNORKELING AND swimming, I didn't feel inspired to run on our small stretch of beach. Nonetheless I ached to explore on dry land, so one morning, I took a ferry to St. John with Stephen and John. We hiked through the national park's leafy jungle to white-sand beaches fronting water the color of sapphires. We swam to Rockefeller's tranquil resort on Caneel Bay and ate an expensive lunch on its terrace, our wet bathing suits and snorkel masks leaving puddles on the smooth tile. Afterward we hiked back to town and devoured two-dollar tacos and margaritas on a deck overlooking Cruz Bay as the sun set and the sky changed from blue to purple and then orange behind the many green islands rising up out of the sea.

But mostly we stayed put, spending time with Taylor in the water or on the beach fronting our resort. When she wasn't swimming, my sister wore a huge straw hat and holed up under a beach umbrella to listen to movies on her portable DVD player. That summer, she'd become more vulnerable to extreme temperatures—just one more consequence of Batten disease. The heat wiped her out, making her lethargic and more susceptible to symptoms like speech problems and even seizures. During the hottest part of the day, we tried to keep her out of the sun.

One afternoon, I brought my lunch to Taylor's chair. Though still a month shy of twelve, she looked like a teenager in her hot pink bikini and painted toenails.

I rummaged through my beach bag and pulled out my camera, then reached over and removed one of my sister's ear buds.

"Hey, T," I said. "You look like you're having a blast. Can I take your picture?"

Taylor obliged by scrunching up her face in a strange, pseudo-smile—something she'd started doing only recently. My sister hadn't seen her own reflection in a long time, I knew. Is it possible to forget how to smile? I supposed it was similar to how, if a person went deaf, their voice could become distorted over time.

I put the camera away without taking Taylor's picture and dug into my salad.

PUNCTUALITY HAS NEVER been a virtue of my family. I remember eating second breakfasts at the bagel shop halfway to our Presbyterian church because Mom and Dad had realized five miles into the longish trip that we weren't going to make it to the sanctuary in time to be seated for the service. So I'd smear cream cheese on fresh bagels, taking care not to stain my Sunday dress, and read verses from the Bible I'd received at confirmation the year I turned nine. We really didn't make it to church that often, but I knew the Bible by heart before I'd finished elementary school.

When I was a kid, the habitual lateness rarely bothered me. One year my father signed up to be our Odyssey of the Mind coach at school. That didn't work out so well, because he often didn't make it to our afterschool practices in the library until a few minutes before the other parents arrived to take my classmates home. In truth, most of us hadn't liked Odyssey of the Mind anyway. We were content playing games or pretending to read books off the shelves whenever the librarian came around, and nobody told their parents that our coach was always late.

But lateness had become a big deal for Taylor recently. Things like medication administration and meals and sleep had to be kept on a tight schedule. And laid-back life in the Virgin Islands didn't fit the complicated logistics of Batten disease.

On our final day, we all tried to squeeze every last drop out of the time we had left. We skimped on breakfast and lunch and spent most of the day outdoors. The temperature rose to over ninety degrees as the unforgiving tropical sun climbed higher in the sky, but nobody wanted to go inside.

"Maybe we should start thinking about dinner," Mom finally said, after the sun had dipped behind a low-hanging cloud.

My mother does not like to go to the grocery store without putting on mascara and a quick swipe of lipstick. But she was the one who suggested we venture out in our bathing suits and cover-ups. After all, it was getting late, and she needed to feed Taylor. Plus, we still had to pack our suitcases after dinner.

So we took a shuttle to a partner resort with more dining options. After some debate, we put our name on the waiting list at a restaurant with tables in an outdoor cabana that caught the breeze off the Caribbean.

We'd just placed our orders when it happened. It was hard to discern much of our surroundings, lit only by soft candlelight on the tables and moonlight on the water, but there was no mistaking the change in my sister's body language. Her head dropped toward her chest, as if she was going to pass out. Then she froze, as if someone had pressed an invisible pause button.

"Taylor? Taylor!" My mother's voice pierced the relative silence in our corner of the restaurant. She touched Taylor's shoulder tentatively. John threw his chair back and stood.

And then, "*Mommy!*" Life flowed back into my sister's limbs. Her sightless eyes darted around the table.

Mom's arms were wrapped around Taylor, who suddenly looked very small. "I don't know what that was, but it scared her," she said.

Then I saw Taylor's face in the dim light, and it dawned on me that she'd had what was probably her first seizure. My sister had just crossed another line.

On the shuttle ride after dinner, John whispered in my ear, "We need to keep her out of the heat as long as possible before we get on the plane tomorrow." When we returned to the hotel, he requested a late checkout while my parents took Taylor, still in a mild state of shock, up to the room.

The lady at the desk shook her head. "I'm sorry, but we can't provide a late checkout."

John leaned forward and lowered his voice, though my family had already gone upstairs. "I'm not asking," he said, not unkindly. "I'm telling."

"Yes, of course," she answered, punching the keys on her computer.

THAT NIGHT, I dreamed I was running barefoot on the beach in front of our resort. I was running near the coral reef where we'd waded with Taylor. I could see the scene clearly—the lush green gardens and white sand that glittered in the sun and water like a thousand liquid jewels. The air tasted pure and clean, my lungs felt full, and my legs felt strong. But I was running in place. No matter how fast I ran, I didn't get anywhere at all.

THE NEXT MORNING, sunlight sparkled like crystals on impossibly blue water beyond the coconut palms lining the beach. A solitary bird rode the morning breeze in one spot, like a kite. Its shadow danced on the emerald and coral roof of the building across the street. I walked onto our private balcony and slid the door shut behind me. It was still early, and it seemed as though no one was stirring but the bird and I. I watched its strange ballet and tried to imagine my sister as a grown woman, snorkeling in the bay or hiking in the tropical forest on St. John or sipping on fancy drinks with little umbrellas at the pool bar.

Taylor will never do those things, I thought. *The seizures won't stop and her speech will get worse and she'll struggle to walk, and then what?* I closed my eyes. I didn't want to think about the future.

Back inside, my family was stirring. Mom had brewed coffee and coaxed my sister and father out of bed and into the small dining area of our villa, where they both sat, their shoulders hunched and their hair mussed. Dad looked the same as he always looked on a weekend morning, but I couldn't take my eyes off Taylor as I fixed my coffee. Something seemed different. The incident at dinner the previous night had changed her. Though she'd gotten nine hours of sleep, she looked wiped out. Her facial features were slack, her spirit dulled.

How long? I wondered as I folded shorts and shirts and bathing suits and tucked them into my suitcase after breakfast. *How much longer will Taylor be able to travel?* I realized with a start that my sister dreamed of going to Hawaii, and we hadn't taken her to Hawaii. *How much longer will she walk?* I thought later as I watched her shuffle through the resort lobby in her Girls on the Run t-shirt, still in a strange, almost comatose state.

In the middle of checkout, my father suggested we take a family picture. We went outside onto one of the balconies so there'd be less commotion and a prettier backdrop. A huge dove-gray cloud had formed over the ocean, and the water looked flat and lifeless—not the beautiful scene from earlier in the morning. But it was great lighting for a picture, I thought. The concierge did the honors.

I didn't look at the photo until we were seated on the plane. In it Dad, Stephen, John, and I are smiling. But Taylor's eyes are cast toward the ground. She seems to be somewhere far away. My mother wears only a half smile, as if the other half couldn't get past the knot of pain. The rain cloud is partly blocking the sun.

The plane's wheels lifted, and the green islands and blue sea faded into a finger-painting far below. For the first time I thought about how, if Taylor wasn't sick, we might not have gone to the Virgin Islands as a family. As the plane soared above the clouds, I closed my eyes for the second time since waking up that morning. In my mind's eye, I saw my sister giggling as clownfish swam circles around her and tickled her feet in the sunlit sea. And somewhere deep inside, I found my silver lining.

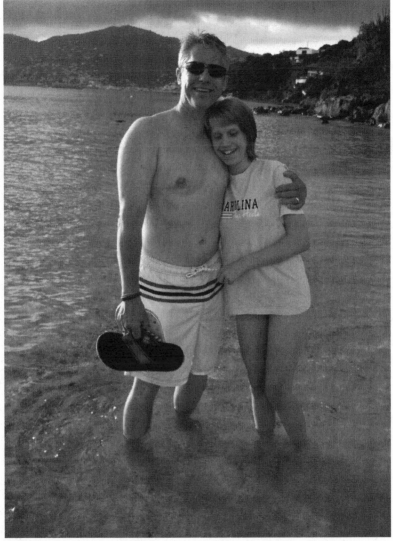

Taylor and her dad on a family trip to the U.S. Virgin Islands, 2010

Chapter 13

TWO WEEKS LATER, I boarded a plane again. On the last Friday in July, heat shimmered off the blacktop in Charlotte, but I'd dressed for air-conditioned hotel meeting rooms and the chilly breeze off Lake Michigan.

I was headed to Chicago to attend the annual Batten Association conference; I traveled solo to give my mother a well-deserved break, since she'd represented us the previous year. I watched cities and lakes and cornfields glide by in miniature far below our plane and tried to steel myself for the next few days. I knew approaching the trip like a job would help me achieve the goals I'd set for my time in Chicago. I knew it'd help me get through the conference in one piece.

But when a cab deposited me on a bustling city street and I walked into the hotel, rolling my suitcase and laptop bag, I felt my shoulders tense up and my mouth go dry. It was my first time attending the conference since I went to Rochester with my mother less than a year after Taylor's diagnosis, and though the place and time had changed, the scene was the same. All around me were families with affected kids in adaptive strollers or wheelchairs. They had vacant eyes, and some of them wore bibs or small towels as drool cloths. A few of the kids yelled unintelligible phrases; their words made it sound as if their tongues were too large and heavy for their mouths.

It didn't seem possible that three years had passed since Mom and I stepped off that escalator into a sea of sick kids in Rochester, and yet I felt as if I'd lived a lifetime. I still remembered the fear I'd felt at the sight of one hundred kids destined to die young. We were so new to the fight then—not quite twelve months removed from the blistering July day when a doctor told my parents my little sister was going to die. I had been scared because I wasn't ready to be part of that world, and seeing it made it real. And yet, I'd had a strange urge to tell everyone at the conference—and maybe everyone on Earth—that my sister would be different. My sister would survive. We were going to save her. I had been raw and innocent and defiant and enormously confident. I had believed without abandon.

But now that attitude seemed reckless, and I was running out of time. So I straightened my back and shoulders, held my head high, and smiled at the families standing by their kids' wheelchairs or camping on overstuffed sofas and chairs as I crossed the hotel lobby and walked toward the front desk to check in.

One thing I'd learned in the four years since the diagnosis was the importance of cherishing each day. At some point I'd figured out that I couldn't tackle Batten disease in chunks of years or months or even weeks. I'd learned how to survive by facing my sister's illness one day at a time. Staring our presumed future in the face for the next several days would be difficult, I knew. But I'd come to Chicago with a mission—to do exactly what I'd said Taylor's Tale would do all along: give Batten disease one hell of a fight. I vowed not to let these days I'd been given go to waste, not to let my fear get the best of me.

I HAD ENJOYED biology as a high school student. I helped my future engineer husband study for tests on subjects like peptide bonds and mitochondria—I can still hear my tenth grade biology teacher championing the powers of "mighty mitochondria"—and I had pictured myself going into exercise science if I could only get over my apprehension about blood and guts. But I always figured I'd be a humanities major in college. I loved T.S. Eliot and F. Scott Fitzgerald more than most teenagers did, and my college roommates sometimes caught me lapsing into Middle English the year I studied the fourteenth-century poem, "Sir Gawain and the Green Knight."

Still, after Taylor's diagnosis I'd slipped into the world of medical doctors and science PhDs with relative ease. They knew I wasn't one of them, but they let me into their circle. Like my mother, I shunned family support sessions, group social outings, and designated free time, instead patching together meetings with handpicked investigators in empty conference rooms or at the quiet end of a crowded bar. I took a pen and paper and scribbled pages of notes about mouse models and drug compounds and project goals.

I walked into my first session in Chicago late Friday afternoon for a research update from several scientists, including Sandy Hofmann. Our board had just approved an additional eighty thousand dollars for Sandy, and even though the Batten Association's scientific advisory board had ranked her proposal highly, I cornered her after the session to probe for more details than she'd shared in her CliffsNotes version for the group.

"How's the work going?" I asked. An eighty thousand dollar question. Sandy looked around the room, as if to make sure there weren't more of me. She closed her laptop and shuffled some papers.

"I need to make some adjustments with the mice, but things are going well. I sent the latest report to the Batten Association," she said.

"What kind of adjustments?"

"Adding proteins to the enzyme to get it across the blood brain barrier," she said. "Trying different injection sites with the mice." Sandy shifted her weight from one leg to the other and stuffed her papers in a bag on the podium.

I already knew that finding a way to get the missing enzyme to the brain was likely our biggest hurdle and that working with mice could be challenging due to their small size and short lifespan. I wanted more details, and I knew Sandy had them in her head. But I could see she was itching to escape. Besides, I said to myself, if I really needed to know the particulars, I'd be more likely to get them if I emailed Sandy later.

And as much as I craved knowledge of lab mice and enzyme production and delivery methods, what I really wanted in that moment was to tell Sandy how grateful I was for her, how I understood there were thousands of other diseases and no one was making her work on Batten disease, and without people like her kids like my sister had no hope. But I had trouble finding the words, and by the time I did, Sandy had muttered a quick goodbye and hurried out of the room, leaving me alone.

THAT NIGHT, A lot of families went to the Cubs game. I'd always wanted to see Wrigley Field's ivy-covered outfield walls in person, but I didn't want to go as a sib—the Batten Association's nickname for siblings of affected children. I was long past denial, but I still hated the label. Like my family's Disney World trip months after the diagnosis, if

I went to Wrigley Field, I'd go on my own terms, without the specter of Batten disease.

Instead of joining the group, I took my laptop to the hotel bar with the intention of writing a blog post and ordered a drink. The rum was cheap and didn't go down smoothly, but it reminded me of the Virgin Islands. I let myself imagine my sister in a scene of sunlight and ocean and gardens. In my mind, Taylor could see.

I was still daydreaming when I got a new email from my sister. She'd recently gotten computer software for the visually impaired that spoke the letters and numbers aloud as she punched the keys. She used it for everything from online music purchases to social studies homework and journaling, which she sometimes did with her teacher for language arts.

journal entry
We went to the virgin islands. John saw a little shark and it ate a fish right in front of his knee. Scary! A BIG iguana sat under my lounge chair. He was as big as sunny with a tail as long as a snake.

"Are you alright?"

I felt the bartender's eyes on me before I looked up from my screen.

"I'm okay," I said, pushing my drink away and rummaging for my wallet. I slid my credit card across the bar and angrily wiped my eyes. I wasn't even sure why I'd gotten upset. Maybe because my sister's email had been so *normal*. Maybe because, if a stranger had read that email, they'd have no idea she was sick, even though she had a brain-wasting disease. Maybe because, if people like Sandy Hofmann couldn't figure things out, kids like my sister would keep dying.

A few researchers I recognized had wandered into the bar, and I pondered putting my laptop away and pulling up a chair. But what I thought I *should* do was not what I *wanted* to do. So I just waved at the table on my way to the lobby, where I took an elevator to my room and changed into shorts and a t-shirt before riding the elevator back down to the bowels of the hotel.

The gym was tiny, with windows or mirrors on all four walls; it reminded me of a terrarium. Not surprisingly for a Friday evening, it was empty. I climbed on the treadmill, and I ran. I tried, unsuccessfully, to run to a place where my sister didn't have Batten disease. But when I crumpled into a heap at the end of my workout, my skin glistening, I was still in the glass box.

I SPENT ALL Saturday morning chasing PhDs, trying to corner them between sessions. Right before lunch, I caught Jonathan Cooper from Kings College London in a hallway crowded with families. I'd always liked Jon; unassuming and kind, he spoke with a charming English accent and shared my love for soccer ("football"). I'd only met him once before, in Rochester, but the Batten world's tight-knit, almost incestuous nature made it easy to stay in touch. Jon was a pathology specialist and collaborated with everyone, so he was a great information source; in fact, he'd be working with Sandy on our project in the upcoming year.

"Can you talk?" I asked, slinging my shoulder bag out of the way to give him a hug.

"Why don't you join us for lunch?" he said, gesturing to a horde of fresh-faced doctoral students from his lab.

I smiled, thinking I'd socialize now and get what I really wanted later. "Sure, that would be great."

Eight of us fixed plates of hotdogs and mystery vegetables—typical lunch fare for a budget-conscious family conference—and found a table near the middle of the banquet hall. Except for Jon, who was in his forties, my tablemates were all exceptionally young. I knew many of them would put in their time with Jon and go on to work on a more high-profile disease after cutting their teeth on the monster killing my sister and the kids at other tables all around us. I hoped at least one of them would stay.

Our conversation bounced from mouse models to drug absorption rates and translational research, with some friendly debate about whether Chelsea would repeat as English Premier League champions in 2011 sprinkled in. I picked at the mushy vegetables on my plate, wishing for fries, and acted the part of the sponge. I had never really thought about how much science I'd learned since Taylor's diagnosis, but I realized then that I understood cell theory almost as well as I understood soccer rules.

I'd always hated my elementary school's science fair. Hated it. I'd had to enter a project every year. But it's not that I hated science. In fact, I found science fascinating long before acing my tenth grade biology class. I'd always felt drawn to science that had a story. I loved learning about planets and galaxies and dreamed of discovering new worlds. As a kid, I had an encyclopedic knowledge of the solar system and dinosaurs and built motorized cars and appliances with the erector set my Granddaddy Parks brought back from F.A.O. Schwarz after one of his trips to New York City. In elementary and middle school, I filled legal pads with science fiction and fantasy stories about alien kidnappers and old mirrors that were gateways to prehistoric worlds.

I always assumed I'd keep writing, and maybe I could use my interest in science in my writing somehow. But I never thought I'd be part of a worldwide effort to fix a rare, fatal childhood disease. I never thought I'd be writing about a disease that was killing my sister. I never thought I'd have to save my little sister's life.

When I looked up from my plate, our group was dispersing. I stood, my hand on the pad and pen I hadn't touched during the meal.

Jon hung back from the others. "I'm sorry we didn't have a chance to chat more. Catch up after the dinner tonight?"

"Yes, that would be great," I said. I gathered my half-eaten lunch and computer bag in a rush, remembering all of a sudden that I was leading one of the afternoon sessions. "I'll be around."

I've got no better place to be, in other words. I didn't come to Chicago to see Chicago. I came to Chicago to save my sister.

THE BATTEN ASSOCIATION did not employ a marketing director, so they'd asked me—a twenty-eight-year-old sibling who'd shunned their sibs program—to lead a session on raising awareness for families and scientists. Before leaving Charlotte, I'd built a PowerPoint presentation and pulled samples of brochures and other Taylor's Tale collateral. Lance and his development director, Adina, hadn't provided any parameters for the talk, so I gave the fifty or so people packed into our meeting room a crash course on everything I'd learned in a six-year marketing career and four years fighting Batten disease, from writing brochure copy to building websites and planning events.

"How can we get our little boy on the news?" one dad asked after I'd gone through my spiel.

I began to tell the man I'd covered that earlier and could talk with him after the session ended, but then I saw his son. A miniature version of his father, with arms and legs that looked as though they'd never been used, he was sleeping in an adaptive stroller. A St. Louis Cardinals cap sat askew on his soft brown hair.

I've been an introvert forever; growing up, the soccer field was the only place I ever got vocal. But vowing I'd do everything to keep Batten disease from killing my sister forced me to face one of my fears—public speaking—and right away, I discovered a knack for it. I could stand in front of five hundred people without seeing any of them. Once I got up there and started talking, it was as if I was alone in the room. It wasn't until after I finished speaking that I saw people's faces. I was good at fooling myself for Taylor.

"Capturing the media and the public's interest is all about having a powerful story," I said, and then, my tone softening, "Your son has a powerful story. You just need to give him a voice."

I felt like I should say something else to the boy's father about press releases and the rules for contacting the media. Then, for the first time, I took in the whole scene in front of me. This wasn't one of our fundraisers. It wasn't a marketing conference or a college classroom. This room was filled with desperate families and dying children and scientists who worked around the clock to save them but hadn't yet succeeded. And when I opened my mouth again, the words wouldn't come. A mother in the front row rescued me by raising her hand to share a story about a dance-a-thon she'd planned in her family's hometown.

"Your presentation was great," Sara said, a blonde woman from Chicago whose little girl had late infantile Batten disease, as I packed up my things a few minutes later. "I learned so much from you. We're starting a website. Would it be okay if I contact you if we have questions?"

"Definitely," I said, handing her my wristband.

A couple whose nametags listed a town outside of Miami stopped by to thank me for the primer on print materials on the way to their next session. A mother from Canada gave me a hug. "We've always wanted to tell our story back home but could never muster the courage," she said.

I'd thought the session hadn't gone well because I faltered at the end. But I had made a difference, despite my inability to answer questions.

SATURDAY AFTERNOON HAD always been designated free time at the Batten Association conference. I was annoyed at myself for not scheduling any meetings with researchers, and I lugged my laptop to the hotel's coffee shop to do penance, even though the sun was shining and I'd packed my running shoes.

I'd brought work from my hospital job because I was behind, and taking time off on Friday hadn't helped. But when I dug into a project for our heart institute, I couldn't focus. In recent months I'd found it tough to be working for a hospital and promoting our ability to heal when we didn't have a damn thing that could help my sister. Pulling results for our ad campaigns and analytics for our website on a regular basis only reminded me that even our patients fighting really terrible things, like congenital heart defects and strokes, had hope in the hands of our doctors and nurses.

But helping out with media events at our children's hospital was the worst. Watching famous athletes play video games or pose for pictures with sick kids while TV cameramen captured the action for the nightly news, I spent as much time worrying the patients would never leave the hospital walls as I did imagining they would get better and go home. The thought of those kids dying young left me heartbroken, while the thought of them conquering leukemia or lymphoma made me angry that Taylor didn't have that luxury.

I hadn't made a dent in my work project before I found myself in danger of crying for the second time since I'd arrived in Chicago. Resigned to the reality that I'd be slammed when I returned to the office on Monday, I packed up my things, went back to my room, and passed out on the freshly made bed.

WHEN IT CAME time to get ready for the banquet that night, I pulled myself together and went downstairs.

The parade of children living with Batten disease was difficult but easier to bear than that first one in Rochester three years earlier; somehow the shock value of dying kids had waned over the past two days in Chicago, and not feeling like I had to protect my mother from so much pain was a huge relief.

I was sitting with a mix of parents and scientists, and during the procession of wheelchairs Mark Sands, a PhD from Washington University in St. Louis, leaned over and whispered in my ear.

"Do you have a few minutes to talk?"

"Right now?" I whispered back. But Mark was already walking toward the back of the darkened room. Realizing I didn't really have the courage to see the rest of those sick kids, I set down my napkin and followed him into the hallway.

Mark was sitting on a bench, his legs crossed at the ankles and his arms loosely crossed over his chest. He had sandy hair and smiled with his eyes, and he wore a plain t-shirt tucked into Wrangler jeans. The first time I'd seen Mark in Rochester, I'd thought he looked more like a rancher than a researcher. We'd helped fund one of Mark's postdoctoral fellows the previous year, and I knew my mother stayed in close touch with him.

Mark motioned for me to sit on the bench next to him. I'd worn heels to dinner and appreciated the invitation.

"What's up?" I dug in my purse for a notepad and pen, all business.

"I hate these things." Mark's head was resting against the wall, and his eyes were closed.

"The conferences?"

"The parades."

I slid the paper back into my purse. "My mom hates them, too. She said she'd never put Taylor on display like that."

"Your mother's a smart woman," Mark said. He opened his eyes. "Listen, I haven't heard from your mom in a while. Can you ask her to drop me a note when you get home?"

"Anything you want to talk about now?"

"Not yet. But hopefully soon."

DURING DESSERT, I presented Sandy with our eighty thousand dollar check. After our stilted exchange in the meeting room earlier I felt more uncomfortable than ever, but I told myself we were supporting the work that had the absolute best chance to save kids with infantile Batten disease. The Batten Association's scientific advisory board apparently agreed, having ranked it at the top of all of the proposals it received.

After the formal program ended, I sipped lukewarm coffee and watched parents and kids flood the small dance floor in the darkened room, and I thought maybe I hated the conference as much as my mother did. I could still hear the defiance in Mom's voice months after my sister's diagnosis. "I didn't ask to join this club," she'd said. She didn't want friendships predicated on a shared tragedy, and she didn't want advice on preparing to lose her child. She just wanted to fix things. I knew that for many families, the annual event was a time to connect with the only other people in the world who could even begin to understand what they were going through, and a time to get advice from clinical experts who could at least attempt to untangle the tangled web of symptoms kids with Batten disease face. While the conference hadn't done those things for me, I'd taken good notes for Taylor's Tale and raised our profile and, I hoped, given other families valuable tools to tell their own stories. I could think of a thousand places I'd rather be, but I thought that when the conference came around again the next year, I'd be there.

Overall, I was glad I had come. But watching the kids in wheelchairs at dinner had made me miss my sister, whose own light was now starting to flicker. I left my half-full coffee cup and slipped upstairs to my room, where I fell into a dreamless sleep, my late meeting with Jon Cooper forgotten.

I took a cab to the airport early Sunday. After boarding the plane, I scrolled through the messages on my phone for the first time that morning and opened a new email with an attachment from Taylor.

Hi laura!
Mommy said you would like this picture. We are hugging on the beach and the sun is shining on the water. I miss you and love you!

It had been waiting for me, calling me home.

Chapter 14

IT'S EASY TO say we'll slow down and make time for the people in our lives; it's another thing altogether to actually do it. "Tomorrow's another day," I'll often say to myself as I watch the minutes and hours tick by and sweat my list of to-do items. I was raised to be a planner. I'm the firstborn daughter of an overachieving mother, and I'm strategic, not spontaneous.

That's why I surprised myself by sending a note to my childhood piano teacher in the fall after I returned from Chicago, even though I hadn't seen or spoken to her in ten years. I'd recently inherited the grand piano that had been my mother's as a teenager, and in my note I explained that I'd started playing again.

Dzidra Reimanis was already sixty years old when I arrived for my first lesson wearing a cotton jumper and pigtails on a balmy summer afternoon not long before I started kindergarten in the mid-1980s. She'd escaped Latvia, a tiny country on the Baltic Sea in northern Europe, in the middle of the night as a young girl. I loved hearing Dzidra's stories and took pride in spelling her name correctly on competition entry forms. She lived with a white cat named Beethoven and owned a mismatched pair of Steinway and Yamaha grand pianos that, positioned back to back, dominated the main area of her small ranch house. Across the street was a pond with ducks and a paved path, and sometimes when my parents were running late after my lesson I'd walk around the lake and watch their graceful landings on the water's smooth surface.

The week after I sent the letter, Dzidra called me. She'd seen stories about my sister in the paper and on television, she said, and she never stopped thinking about us. Would I join her for breakfast one morning before work? I said yes, and after meeting her at a neighborhood diner on my way to the office the next day, I wondered why I'd let so many years pass between visits. This woman who had been present for so much of my childhood was eighty-three years old, and one day soon I'd drive by the ranch house by the pond with the ducks and she'd be gone, I realized—a terrible thought to have over pancakes.

After reconnecting with Dzidra, I understood more than ever that my time with Taylor, too, was limited. I made a real effort to do more things with my sister, because I knew I couldn't take her for granted. I took her tubing on the lake and reveled in her roller coaster screams. We played the bowling and hula-hoop and karaoke games on her video game system; when she sang the karaoke songs, I noticed she'd stopped singing all of the lyrics, instead hanging on individual notes for a long time. We baked homemade pizzas and plunked the keys on my piano after washing the pizza grease from our hands. We watched movies like *The Sound of Music* until Taylor fell asleep on my sofa in her pink pajamas and fuzzy pink socks.

But even in the happiest moments I could feel the anger burning in my chest. Why *couldn't* we take these things for granted? Why couldn't Taylor paddle the kayak with her younger cousins? Why did she have to stay with an adult at the age of twelve? Why couldn't she see the pins fall when she bowled a strike? Why did a girl who loved to sing have to suffer from speech problems? *Why?*

Before Batten, I'd assumed I'd always have my sister around, and I missed a lot of the beauty all around me. So I understood why other people missed things in their own lives. Sometimes we don't appreciate soccer games and ballet recitals and school plays as long as we think next week will bring more of the same. I tried to feel grateful that I'd gotten a wake-up call to pay attention and be present. But it never worked, and I was still angry as hell at Batten disease.

Instead of getting mad, Taylor embraced her challenges.

"I get to walk to class with friends," she told me one night when we were curled up on the loveseat in my bonus room in front of a cartoon.

"What do your friends do?"

"They help me. So I don't get lost."

"Who are some of your friends? Who helps you?" I asked.

"My girlfriends. And Mr. Swistak walks with me sometimes. He's nice."

It occurred to me then that at Taylor's age, walking to class with an adult probably would have embarrassed me. But Fletcher serves kids with learning disabilities, and all of my sister's classmates were dealing with one challenge or another—even if Taylor represented an extreme. They went through normal growing pains like all preteens, but walking my sister to class just didn't strike them as weird. On some level, the kids thought it was cool; they all wanted to be her walking buddy. And while she didn't like being different, I think Taylor was so good at taking her struggles in stride that her classmates respected her. They wouldn't have dared tease her.

"Who is Mr. Swistak?" I asked.

"He fixes the computers and he teaches the boys running."

Andrew, I thought. Andrew Swistak, The Fletcher School's IT director, who also coached the boys' track and cross country teams. I'd seen him across the school cafeteria at some of the talent shows and other events on campus, and I thought maybe he'd been at Taylor's first race. I smiled down at my sister curled up in the crook of my arm. She had a silly grin on her face, like she was imagining how the boys in her class would look wearing short track shorts.

But as upbeat as she was, my sister wasn't invincible. Since the start of the school year she'd noticed some of the changes to her body—normal changes most girls her age experienced, like developing breasts and her first period—yet changes that were difficult and awkward because she was blind and needed more help. To make things worse, the creeping shadow of Batten disease had started stealing other things besides her vision. Sometimes she'd stumble over her words or repeat words, particularly if she got excited. She'd been a firecracker as a little kid, but lately she'd become a little more withdrawn and reclusive; it was easy for her to become over-stimulated in a noisy place or new environment. We'd go to a loud pizza place or basketball game, and all of a sudden she'd shut down. She'd have to work so hard to process the commotion that she couldn't respond to us.

I think my sister's preteen and early teen years were the toughest for her, because they marked that intersection of time when she started to lose ground more quickly but was still sharp enough to pick up on the fact that it was happening. As a result, she grew scared and depressed on top of the normal crap every girl that age endures. Her body was failing her, and now her mind was failing her, too. But despite her cognitive struggles, Taylor remained clever. In those days she was always more aware of the situation than most people thought. Also with the loss of her vision, her hearing had improved, as if to pick up the slack. But a lot of people assumed that because she was blind, they could talk about her when she was around. They'd whisper about her, and she'd pick up on it because she was hypersensitive to it. She'd tilt her head toward a conversation; that's how I knew when she was listening. I'd watch her expression change as she heard people talk about some activity they were going to enjoy and then figured out that she wouldn't be part of it.

My sister's emotional health was, in turn, impacting my emotional health. I didn't cry as much as before, but a deep sadness had set in by the time the first leaves changed in October. I couldn't shake it. I was tired all the time. Even if I went to bed at a decent hour, I strained to swing my legs out of bed at the sound of my alarm in the morning. I'd always had headaches, but they were getting out of control.

I'd become proficient at holding it all inside. But when I couldn't bear it anymore, I lost it at my hair salon, of all places.

The salon assistant, Dinah, swept wavy gold locks into a dustpan while the stylist, Debbie, swiped my credit card at the front desk. I was the salon's last customer of the evening, and streetlights twinkled outside.

"Can I ask you something?" Dinah set the broom against the textured wall and wiped her hands.

I looked up at her reflection in the full-length mirror. "Sure."

"What is your sister's prognosis?"

What was I supposed to say? I'd often gotten that question but rarely gave an honest answer. I could always tell when friends were afraid of how I'd respond. Tragedy is naturally uncomfortable for people. A lot of people *want* to be there for you, but their support is conditional; when really bad stuff is involved, they're scared to death they'll have to bear part of your pain.

I'd come to expect variations of the question, so I'd created several stock responses over the years. I refused to give the hopeless romantics what they wanted, which was the impossible: *Taylor is doing much better!* or *We're out of the woods!* or *The surgery/medicine worked! She's all better now! Can you believe it? We can't either! But we'll roll with it!* This was Batten disease, after all. And the only thing I knew for sure about Batten disease was that no child had ever survived it. They all traveled their own road, but all roads led to the same end. I couldn't say that, though; people have enough misery in their own lives without shouldering ours, too. So while I refused to make Batten sound better than it is, I still felt the need to be positive. *She's a fighter!* I'd say—which was true; or: *We've made amazing progress for kids like her!* That was true, too, though I only said it on days when I really didn't want to talk about Taylor.

But something in Dinah's eyes that night at the salon made me realize she didn't want a stock response. She hadn't asked because she wanted to feel better about the world but because she really wanted to *know*.

Debbie joined us before I could answer.

"I was just asking Laura about her sister," Dinah said.

Debbie had a bag on her shoulder and a ring of keys in her hand. "Don't worry," she said as I watched her set both on the counter. "We've got time. How *is* Taylor?"

Suddenly I was spilling my guts, all of that pent-up anger came tumbling out, and before I knew it both Debbie and Dinah were red-eyed. Thirty minutes later, I didn't have anything else to say. The rush hour traffic on the street below had dwindled to a few cars. Debbie had declared that she'd already cried a little and didn't want to cry a lot, and she couldn't do that in front of me, so why didn't we all just head out?

A light rain began to fall as I drove home. I kept a tight grip on the wheel, but my mind wandered as I watched fat droplets collect on the windshield. The road that had been packed with cars when I'd taken it to work that morning stretched out before me, empty and shining where the glow of the traffic lights mixed with rain and motor oil stains.

I don't know if I can pinpoint the exact moment my perspective on the fight to save my sister started to change. I don't remember coming to the realization that Batten disease was bigger than us, no matter how brave my sister seemed. But somehow, watching the rain fall from the sky, I started to understand that *I* had changed, and that just as Taylor would likely never regain the gifts she'd lost, I would never get back to a truly safe place again. In the beginning, I'd just wanted to fight, fight, fight. I was a woman on a mission. I told anyone who would listen that we'd save my sister. As if buying a cure for Batten disease was as easy as going to the local pharmacy and picking up a prescription. As if I could wave a magic wand, and Taylor would be able to see again, and I'd help her with homework and go to her swim meets and school plays and life would be normal. But as time went on, I lost that early confidence. I winced when my sister struggled with her speech or lost her way in an unfamiliar room. I hadn't really accepted my sister's lot—at least not yet.

Denial seemed so much easier. But it was hard to keep the monster at bay. Though I didn't like to think about it, deep down I understood we were running out of time. And one day, I started saying "kids like Taylor" instead of "Taylor" whenever I talked about the research we supported.

LUCKILY FOR TAYLOR'S Tale, my mother was holding it together. In November, she traveled to Bethesda, outside of Washington, D.C., for a scientific workshop organized and sponsored by other families fighting infantile and late infantile Batten disease.

The small town of Bethesda, Maryland, is one of the most highly educated communities in the nation, making it a natural choice for a meeting of experts on whom we were depending to fix Batten disease. The regulars from past Batten Association and Lysosomal Disease Network meetings, like Sandy Hofmann and Jon Cooper and Mark Sands, were there. But when Mom called me the night she returned home, she couldn't stop talking about a junior investigator from a lab just two hours up the road, at the University of North Carolina Gene Therapy Center.

"Steve Gray is young. He can't be much older than you. But Laura, you wouldn't believe some of the things he's doing. He's been working on a disease called GAN for two years. There aren't even one hundred kids in the whole world with GAN. So no one was working on it before a little group like ours called Hannah's Hope started funding Steve's lab. Now Steve is doing things that have never been done before, and they could make it to trial in a few years. And he's focused on *translational* research. He only cares about saving kids."

"Would he work on Batten—"

"He would, if we funded it. I think we wait and watch the GAN work, at least for right now. But we need to learn more."

Suddenly I remembered a gene therapy trial that had already happened at Cornell—not for Taylor's form of the disease, but for late infantile Batten, its close cousin. I had a fuzzy image of meeting the head of the trial, a doctor with a short stature and a scowl; at the time I'd struggled to imagine him at the bedside of a sick child.

"How would this be different from what Dr. Crystal did in New York?" Dr. Crystal. I was sure that was his name. The Batten community loved him; he'd been treated almost like a celebrity at the two conferences I'd attended.

"Different vector and delivery method," Mom said without hesitation, like she'd expected the question.

"What's a vector?"

"It's what they use to carry the corrected gene to cells." I heard suitcase zippers being zipped shut and the clatter of metal hangers on closet rods. "Listen, I'll explain it all later. I'm too tired for more than basic science."

"So what's next?" I asked, somehow knowing my mother already had a plan.

"We meet with Steve here, in North Carolina. We ask good questions. And we chart our next move."

"Did you talk about getting together?"

"Mark your calendar," she said. "We're having dinner the first week of January."

"You work quickly."

"These kids aren't getting any better," my mother replied. "We need to get going."

THE IMPENDING MEETING with the investigator from North Carolina gave me hope, but I still couldn't shake the funk that had wrapped me up and shut out all the light. I wanted—needed—to run more than ever. I needed to run as a way to expel all of the pent-up anger and nervousness that had built up inside.

I was set to run my second half marathon at Thunder Road ten days before Christmas. On a Sunday afternoon in early December, I drove to the YMCA in a cold, pouring rain to train on the indoor track suspended above the basketball courts. I hit the small oval with my heart set on completing one hundred twenty laps—ten miles.

I coasted for the first few miles as I waited for my muscles to get warm. Near the end of the third mile, it occurred to me that I'd run nearly the distance of one of my sister's 5Ks. I came around the bend and lifted my head. The water fountains were at the end of the straightaway. I thought about how Taylor never saw the finish lines she crossed. I'd sprint when the finish line of a race came into view, but Taylor had to get her energy from somewhere else. Somewhere deep down.

Two laps into my fourth mile, I got a bad cramp, like someone was twisting an invisible knife in my side. I let my mind wander, hoping the physical pain would subside. I thought about how, if I were Taylor, I'd be running in darkness. I was too scared to try it on one of the turns, but I closed my eyes for an instant on one of the straight sections. Right away I felt other people around me on the small track and knew I wouldn't make it to the far end without a collision. On the elevated track, I could feel every person's footfall. It seemed as if the rubber surface beneath my feet was moving, and suddenly I imagined slamming into one of the columns or aluminum advertisement displays that lined the walls. I opened my eyes, shaken.

I'd only completed half of my workout. But after my failed attempt at blind running, I knew I was done. I walked to my car in the rain, not even bothering to open the umbrella in my bag. I was tired, and as I slid behind the wheel with aching muscles, I wondered why, after an injury-filled soccer career, not a cross-country career, I'd decided to become a distance runner. But I knew the answer.

I'd become a distance runner—if not a good one—because of my sister. I knew that the following Saturday, I'd cross the finish line of my second half marathon, even if I had to crawl. I knew I could never stop running. Quitting wasn't Taylor's style. I'd had a tough year, but quitting wasn't my style, either.

A GRAY PALLOR hung over the city on the morning of the Thunder Road race, and a bitter wind cut through my sweatshirt and wicking top. I huddled with my friends Amy and Parker in the throng of humans gathered behind the start line, clapping my hands together and hoping for body heat.

Shortly after the race began, Amy reached out and tapped me on the shoulder. "Look," she said, her breath making a tiny white cloud in the freezing cold. She pointed at a man in a blue fleece who was running a few yards away from us. It took me a second to figure out he was running with a cane. He was blind.

Seconds later I lost the blind runner—and my friends—in the crowd.

Runners, even world-class ones, can do a lot of thinking in the time it takes to run 13.1 miles. As the crowd thinned and I settled into my stride, I was pleasantly surprised to find that I felt fit enough to let my mind wander and keep up a good pace, especially after my disastrous last training run. Soon the landscape of office buildings and houses and trees became so fuzzy that I could have been running anywhere. And for the first time in months, I saw our fight against Batten disease—and in a way my entire life—with perfect clarity.

Maybe it's the same for anyone facing a crisis, but I was tired of being angry. I was tired of being sad. I thought about how I'd cried all the time when we first learned Taylor was sick. Somewhere along the way, my life before Batten disease dropped out of sight in the rear-view mirror. I cried less and less. By then, I mostly just stayed angry. Anger could be good in a way, because it made me want to fight like hell. I thought that sadness wouldn't get me anywhere. But the sadness was still there, even if I'd gotten better at keeping it inside. And when I felt it creep into the corners of my eyes, I ran if possible.

I love running because it makes me feel powerful, I thought as I neared mile ten. *Each time my ruined feet and ankles pound against the pavement, I beat back the tide. Mostly, it's working.* Right then, my head told me to quit the race as my injured joints screamed for mercy. But I kept running.

Thousands of runners were on the course that morning. I couldn't have found my friends Amy and Parker again if I'd tried. Nonetheless for some reason, I crossed paths with the blind runner not once, but twice on our shared journey, as we ran underneath a bridge together less than a mile from the finish line. I can't say the same about any other runner in the field with any degree of certainty. I'm not really superstitious. But I believe in divine intervention.

I'd made it that far because I was running for my sister. And when I saw the blind runner under the bridge, I knew Taylor was right there with me. A few minutes later, the finish line came into view. Taylor helped me find my wings, and I sprinted the rest of the way.

Chapter 15

I WAS RAISED to be a fighter: to work hard, to accept nothing less than the very best from myself. It's in my blood.

I remember riding the bench on my high school soccer team as a freshman. During games I sat by the water cooler, the eyes of the parents and siblings and boyfriends scattered throughout the metal bleachers burning holes in the back of my jersey that always stayed clean. That year my grandparents drove six hours round-trip for nearly every game, even though we played on weeknights and they owned and managed two businesses and I rarely got onto the field. I'd come in with high expectations of myself. So when I didn't play, the vulnerable, scared girl in me wanted to give up. Better to run away than be embarrassed, I thought.

But Grandma Kathryn encouraged me to stick it out. She taught me to hold my head high, even if the coach didn't think I was one of the eleven best players on the team. She didn't know much about soccer, but she was so good that deep down I wanted to make her proud. Whenever I didn't want to jog in the rain or work on my footwork after school, I could hear her gentle encouragement in the back of my head. By my junior year, I was a livewire and one of our most vocal leaders on the field, and I didn't sit on the bench anymore. After playing every minute of a double-overtime win against our archrival in my last season and graduating as our assists leader, I remember thinking that good things come to those who wait, but also to those who work.

My mother is a lot like *her* mother. And instead of wallowing in the misery of Batten disease, she attacked it, even as Taylor's condition worsened. I was the president of Taylor's Tale in name, but she was the one carrying us. I'd finished Thunder Road on a high note, but then winter had come and the darkness and cold had enveloped me and I was spiraling toward a dark place different than anything I'd felt before.

I took my cues from Mom. On a Tuesday night in early January, I watched a jungle of billboards and green exit signs whizz past my window as she drove us to Greensboro, where my Uncle David lived.

The town is ninety miles northeast of Charlotte and a short distance from Chapel Hill, where the junior investigator Steve Gray had worked at the University of North Carolina Gene Therapy Center since getting his PhD from Vanderbilt in 2006. David wasn't on call at the hospital that night, and he'd agreed to have dinner with us so he could help translate the details of Dr. Gray's research on the ultra-rare childhood disease giant axonal neuropathy, or GAN, for the rest of our board.

"I have a good feeling about this," Mom said as she maneuvered around an eighteen-wheeler. "Did you know that the GAN work could be ready for clinical trial in a few years?"

"Can you explain what Dr. Gray is doing, again?" I asked.

"He's taking a healthy copy of the gene and packaging it in a viral vector," she said. "The vector takes the good copy of the gene to the cells that need it. Like a delivery truck."

I stared at my mother. In another life, she'd been a piano teacher. Now she knew viral vectors like she'd once known Beethoven's Ninth Symphony.

STEVE GRAY WAS waiting for us when we arrived at the restaurant a few miles off the interstate. I'd seen photos of him on the Hannah's Hope website and picked him out in a booth near the back of the room.

"You were right—he's young," I whispered to Mom as we walked behind the hostess toward the table.

"Just wait," Mom whispered back, and then, "I don't care if he's sixteen. He's the one."

Steve stood and extended a hand when we approached. He had a slight build and a face that looked as if it'd never known a razor. Beneath a shock of brown hair, he had kind eyes that immediately made me feel relaxed.

"Good to see you again, Sharon," he said. "You must be Laura," he said to me, shaking my hand. He smiled. "I heard a lot about you at the workshop in Bethesda."

"I hope it was all good," I joked, sliding into the booth beside my mother.

The excitement with which Mom had first talked about meeting the gene therapy expert in Bethesda carried into our conversation that

January night, but Steve was soft-spoken and unassertive. In fact, at first he mostly asked about Taylor and talked about Hannah Sames, the kinky-haired little girl from upstate New York whose parents, Lori and Matt, had raised millions of dollars for a disease no one had ever heard of. In less than two minutes, I'd learned that like Taylor, Hannah loved singing and dancing as much as she loved playing outdoors and that she had an affinity for strange foods, like pickles for breakfast.

"Getting to know the kids we're fighting to save is important to me," Steve said. He leaned across the table to show me a photo of the little girl on his phone. She had bright eyes and a big smile framed by tightly coiled, strawberry blonde hair. "The doors of our lab are decorated with pictures like this," he added. "Seeing the faces of the kids fighting the diseases we study every day is a constant source of motivation. It makes it a lot easier to come in on a Saturday if I know it'll get us closer to saving the Hannahs of the world."

Half of the three hundred fifty million people affected by a rare disease are children, and a lot of those rare diseases, like GAN and Batten disease, are fatal. It occurred to me that Steve and his lab mates were in the business of saving kids whose families had been told they didn't have a shred of hope. After that night when my mom first returned from the meeting in Bethesda, I'd forgotten to ask her more about what made Steve Gray's brand of gene therapy so different from Ron Crystal's at Cornell. Some people in the research world might have wondered why we were so gung-ho about Steve when Dr. Crystal had already done so much with Batten disease. But from the moment I met Steve, something about the precocious PhD who'd arrived in my home state the same summer my sister was diagnosed just made me believe. I couldn't explain it.

We'd only just ordered drinks when Uncle David appeared. He looked sharp in an expensive dress shirt and tie, so I knew he'd spent the afternoon in his clinic rather than the operating room. He exchanged quick hellos with Steve and sat down.

Steve gave us a primer on GAN. The effects of the ultra-rare disease are similar to ALS, but it starts in early childhood. A protein called gigaxonin malfunctions in children with GAN, causing tightly packed, swollen "giant" axons. This disturbs communication between the central nervous system and peripheral nervous system. Kids like Hannah have trouble walking. They can also lose their sense of touch, motor coordination, strength, and reflexes. Hearing and vision can be impaired, too. Kinky hair, like Hannah's, is common among kids with GAN. Most patients don't live past their early twenties, so for Hannah, her family's quest was a race against time. It sounded all too familiar.

Hannah's Hope had begun funding Steve's research on GAN in the fall of 2008, two years earlier. Over appetizers, Steve described how a viral vector—a delivery truck, like my mother had said earlier—could transport a healthy copy of the GAN gene to nerve cells. In theory, he said, they could correct the disease with a one-time treatment—a far cry from the expensive, lifelong enzyme replacement therapy approach we'd been funding since the summer after Taylor's diagnosis.

As Steve talked, I realized my mother the piano teacher—not my uncle the neurosurgeon—was the one asking most of the questions. David was polite and once asked for more details about the delivery method, but Mom's questions came in waves, and by the time our dinner arrived, I could see that she knew a lot more about GAN than most doctors. I couldn't expect David to be an expert on a disease he'd never seen in his clinic, but Mom's passion for beating Batten had given her the ability to soak up science like a sponge.

The gene therapy prodigy ducked out after dinner to put his young children to bed, but Mom and I stood in the parking lot talking to David long after Steve's taillights disappeared around the bend.

"Steve Gray is the real thing," my mother said.

"He's doing good work," David agreed. "And I've heard good things about gene therapy." He paused. A cold breeze blew through the naked branches of the trees by the quiet street, and I felt the hairs on my arms rise beneath my thin jacket.

"But it's probably at least a decade away from helping kids like Taylor, Sharon," David went on, his voice suddenly detached. "Enzyme replacement is further along and more likely to be clinically relevant before gene therapy. Plus, think about how far we've come with Sandy. She's your best advocate and hope."

Mom nodded slowly. Whereas moments earlier she'd been ready to put our money on gene therapy, I could tell David's skepticism had dulled her earlier enthusiasm. He was a doctor, after all; didn't he know better? But on the other hand, David wasn't fighting this war in the trenches, and she was. My uncle had a medical degree, but my mother went to all of the conferences and read all of the literature and lived the battle against Batten disease every day. She got a look on her face like she was thinking hard, her jaw set in the parking lot's harsh lighting even as she stretched to hug her little brother's six-three frame.

"Thanks for coming," she said softly. "Thanks for helping us fight for Miss T."

MY MIND WAS racing with questions I wanted to ask my mother, but I was quiet as we sped past truck stops and fast food restaurants en route to Charlotte. Instead, as we passed the exit for the tiny house where my grandparents now lived a few miles from David and Holly's house, I thought about the Lewy body dementia ravaging Grandma Kathryn. Steve had said that the gene therapy treatment approach could potentially work for lots of diseases besides GAN—not only Batten disease but also Lewy body dementia, Alzheimer's disease, ALS, and a wide range of metabolic diseases, plus many more. I knew we were probably too late to save my grandmother. But after fighting an ultra-rare disease like Batten disease for four-plus years, my pulse quickened when I imagined the possibilities of a treatment with the potential to easily translate to many diseases. I knew more people would listen to us if the science we supported could have a direct impact on them or someone they loved.

Now, when I looked back on the months leading up to my grandmother's diagnosis in 2008, I recognized the signs. But at the time I'd attributed her occasional odd comments and vacant facial expressions to depression stemming from Taylor's diagnosis. My grandmother's children and grandchildren were everything to her; I think the thought of Taylor dying young might have killed her if the Lewy body dementia wasn't already devastating her brain and clouding her understanding of Taylor's disease—a minor blessing.

Grandma Kathryn had always taught me that it was important for us to experience hardship. "Adversity makes you strong," she'd said to me once when I was struggling with depression as a college freshman.

But now two of the people I loved most were losing their battles to brain disease, and as we pulled into my driveway, I felt sure this wasn't what Grandma Kathryn had meant when she encouraged me to embrace adversity. I hugged my mother goodnight and walked inside, my mind still bursting with unanswered questions and my fear of the future tightening its grip.

I DON'T KNOW what I was expecting, but we didn't immediately write a check to kick-start gene therapy for Batten disease under Steve Gray. Mom called it watchful waiting, though I knew David had influenced her hesitation. But when it came time to renew grants that summer we didn't fund anyone else, either, and while she didn't say it, I think my mother's grand plan was to put away money for Steve until everyone else wizened up.

Meanwhile, I tried to focus on supporting Taylor's Tale and keeping my own head above water. I returned to Chapel Hill to run the Tar Heel 10 Miler for Taylor in April and shaved twelve minutes off my previous time. I spoke at six fundraisers in the first half of the year; at one, a college basketball tournament viewing party at a local watering hole, a woman I'd never met walked up to me, squeezed my arm, looked into my eyes, and asked, "Is she going to be okay?"

Taylor was less than ten feet away but clearly wrapped up in her own private, dark world. She sat slumped in my parents' booth, fingering a ball of soft putty that her physical therapist said would help with some of the neuropathy in her hands.

"We still believe in miracles," I said without flinching. I figured that was true, and I didn't feel like getting into the particulars with my sister sitting within earshot.

I knew it wasn't the answer the woman wanted, but it made me think about other miracles I'd witnessed lately. Checks from random strangers arriving in the Taylor's Tale mailbox. Taylor running up the stairs to answer the phone when we didn't think she could do that anymore. Three different boys dancing with my sister at the recent Fletcher School dance. Miracles, I was learning, came in many different forms.

I HADN'T BROKEN my habit of late nights and weekends on the computer, but I made sure to relish my time with Taylor. One Saturday night I offered to watch her so my parents could celebrate a friend's birthday. We baked a homemade pizza with fresh pizza dough; Taylor placed the pepperonis, and the end result tasted delicious, even if the toppings were lopsided.

"Do you want to watch a movie, T?" I asked after dinner, reaching across the table to wipe some of the pizza sauce from my sister's chin.

"*Ella Enchanted*," she said after taking a few seconds to process my question.

When I was twelve, I wouldn't have watched a movie like *Ella Enchanted* even if my parents tied me down. I would have figured out a way to escape or, if that didn't work, squeezed my eyes shut and stuck my fingers in my ears. At that age, I wore cutoff denim shorts and t-shirts, and my most prized possessions were my *Legend of Zelda* Nintendo game (Stephen wasn't allowed to touch it) and the black and orange Nike cleats that matched my middle school soccer jersey.

I loved hanging out with my girly sister in spite of our differences. I appraised the outfit she'd chosen—a frilly cotton shirt and cotton skirt, with sparkly earrings. In that moment it was easy to imagine counseling her on boy problems and taking her to visit colleges and helping her plan her wedding.

"We can watch *Ella Enchanted*," I said. "Go pull it out, and I'll be right there." Taylor's vision teacher had helped her label all of her DVDs in braille, and she'd quickly learned how to find the movie she wanted. But the skills she'd worked so hard to develop were already fading. I knew there was a good chance she'd have to ask me for help. While my sister thumbed through her massive movie collection, I counted out nine pills from the various bottles on the counter and carried them into the family room with a glass of water.

"Here's Ella," Taylor said, handing me an electric blue disc decked out in glitter and stars and a thin strip printed with raised braille dots. I grinned as I saw she'd gotten it right.

"I'll trade you," I said. "We'll watch the movie if you take your pills."

My sister nodded and put out her hand; she didn't like to be fed, because it made her feel like a baby. So we stood in front of my parents' fireplace where she used to give private concerts, and she dutifully took all nine of those pills without saying a word. I couldn't help but think how we couldn't escape Batten disease, even on something as simple as movie night.

As much as I loved my sister, I didn't share her love for Ella, and my mind wandered a few minutes into the movie. The fight against rare disease is a bitch, I thought. Taylor's spunk was like nothing I'd ever seen, but it was hard to watch her struggle with pizza decorating and then pop pills instead of candy. I'd made a pact with myself to not be angry about our situation, but it was hard not to be angry when I had so much hatred for Batten disease and everything it represented. I hated it for all it had stolen from Taylor and all I knew it'd steal from her in the weeks and months and years to come. And yet somehow, through all that hate, I still found happiness in the most unusual places, like cockeyed homemade pizzas and princess movies.

I could sense good things happening in our battle afield, too.

I thought about the kinky-haired, sweet-faced Hannah Sames and her strong-willed mother, Lori. I thought about their boy star Steve Gray, who had arrived in North Carolina the same year my sister was diagnosed with Batten disease. I thought about how, barely two years before, Hannah's parents had asked Steve to find an answer for GAN—like Batten disease, a monster that affects relatively few children worldwide. I thought about how our odds of succeeding when Taylor's Tale had first gotten started seemed insurmountable. But all signs pointed to a clinical trial for GAN in the not-too-distant future, all because one family wasn't willing to take "no cure" for an answer. I thought that maybe one day soon, because families like Hannah's and mine believed and scientists like Steve Gray showed up at the lab each day driven by the faces of kids on their hallway doors, kids like Hannah and my sister wouldn't have to lose their lives to an orphan disease.

Chapter 16

DURING THE LAST game of the women's league season, on a balmy April night, my left Achilles popped and I had to crawl from the soccer field to my car. The doctor at the urgent care center put my injured leg in a walking boot, where it stayed for the rest of the spring and most of that summer. The tendon hadn't ruptured, but I was unable to run and spent a lot of time swimming laps instead.

Throughout those long stretches in the pool when I couldn't listen to music and the scenery never changed, I thought a lot about where Taylor's Tale was headed. As a runner who avoided treadmills in favor of the freedom offered by the outdoors, I disliked the monotony of swimming. I counted my laps but felt as if I was stuck in neutral, and in a way I felt like Taylor's Tale was stuck in neutral, too. Sandy Hofmann and the other Batten experts hadn't submitted new grant requests that summer, but Mom and I had somehow agreed to delay funding for Steve Gray's Batten disease work without ever discussing it. Sometimes I remembered talking to Mark Sands in Chicago and told myself I'd ask my mother what had come of his work, but I never did. Meanwhile, Hannah's Hope kept working fundraising miracles, and Steve continued to speed toward the world's first clinical trial for GAN.

As my recovery dragged, I grew more and more frustrated. Two months became three. It felt as if I'd been injured for an eternity, and I hated not being able to run. Running wasn't just something I did for my sister. I knew my feet couldn't carry Taylor out of the darkness, but running gave me another vehicle to tell her story, and it cleared my head. It was a lot cheaper than counseling and massages and exotic vacations, and I felt sure it had contributed its fair share to my survival over the years. I'd become addicted to running, something even more clear to me now that I couldn't have it. Each night when I got home, I wanted to peel off the wretched boot and stuff it into the trash.

Taylor liked the boot, though. "I can write my name," she said one day while we were eating bowls of ice cream in my kitchen. "Like on Rachel's." Taylor's friend Rachel had sprained her arm that year and had worn a cast. All of the kids at school had written their names in marker on the pink plaster; it was easy to pick out my sister's name when I saw Rachel at a school function because the letters were so crooked.

"You can't write on this, sweetie," I told her. "It's black polyester and plastic. Like a robot leg." Taylor giggled. She reached down toward where my "robot" boot was resting on the floor. She wanted to touch it. "Here," I said, taking her hand. It was sticky with melted vanilla ice cream. "Feel it?" I ran the tips of her sparkly pink polished fingers along the boot's plastic sides and Velcro straps and knocked the boot's hard sole against the tiled floor. She laughed at the clunky sound it made.

That was the thing about Taylor. She could always find something good in the bad. Here she was, blind and struggling to hold a spoon. And yet store-brand ice cream and an orthopedic walking boot made her happy as could be. She acted like everything was right with the world. But of course that wasn't true. I knew my Achilles would heal, but that didn't matter when I also knew Taylor wouldn't.

MY FIRST DAY of freedom from the robot boot fell on the last Thursday in July. Two days after getting clearance from my doctor, John and I flew to Seattle and took a ferry to the town of Port Angeles, then drove our rental car to a mountainous area called Hurricane Ridge in Olympic National Park. Clumps of evergreen trees dotted lingering blankets of snow and cascaded down lush green slopes. Blacktail deer grazed in meadows brushed with wildflowers under an aqua sky.

We'd planned the trip for months. I'd handled all the arrangements, even though it had been John who insisted I needed to get away from Charlotte and get lost in the wilderness for a while. "You need to go to a place where Batten's not in your face," he'd said, telling me he didn't care how long we stayed or how much it cost as long as it made me happy. I knew he was right. I knew I needed to take a break from managing volunteers and a website and writing my blog and watching my sister get sicker on top of all of the stressors that were normal for most people, like work deadlines and paying for our kitchen renovation.

It worked, mostly. I remember watching the sun glisten like liquid gold on a glacial lake and "skiing" down the snow-packed hiking trails of Mount Rainier in our hiking boots and imagining what it would be like if John and I never went home. But one night before dinner I was lying on my back on the picnic table outside our cabin in the remote North Cascades, watching the sky, and I thought about how my dad taught me to look for pictures in the clouds when I was a little girl, and I hated Batten because Taylor couldn't do that anymore.

WE FLEW HOME on the twelfth day, and reality returned with a vengeance. We'd caught the redeye to Charlotte because it was cheaper, and I've never been able to sleep on planes. John took a nap after breakfast, but with our luggage and my laptop and file folders in plain sight, I couldn't stand the thought of being idle. I emptied our suitcases and washed our grimy hiking clothes and scrubbed dirt from the forests of the Pacific Northwest off our scuffed suede and Gore-Tex boots. On the second load of laundry, I sat down at the kitchen table with a cup of coffee and started tackling emails.

By afternoon I was editing the photos from Washington on my laptop when I felt a sudden, sharp pain behind my left eye, as if someone had stuck my brain with a hot poker. Blood pulsated beneath my temples. The acoustic guitar playing on the radio sounded like a screaming fire engine and the sunlight streaming through the window blinded me and the cotton shirt on my back felt like chainmail. My hands flew to my head, and like a deranged person I dug my fingers into my scalp. I felt like I couldn't breathe.

The migraine ravaged my exhausted brain. When John found me I was writhing on the floor, my vision blurry and my speech slurred. I vaguely remember him carrying my limp body to the car, strapping me into the passenger seat, and driving me to the emergency room. Lying in the hospital bed, I thought maybe I was dying.

Death had always been a stranger to me. My Granddaddy Parks had succumbed to a weak heart the winter I was fourteen, but I was in Georgia at a soccer tournament the weekend he took his last breath; when I got home, there was just an empty bed, the sheets washed and folded and put away, so I never had to say goodbye. Because he'd died while I was away, it was easy to imagine that my grandfather, who'd traveled all over the world, was simply on a long trip. Then a year after Taylor was diagnosed, my great-grandmother, for whom Taylor was named, passed away in her sleep. At the viewing I hung toward the back of the funeral home parlor. "Don't you want to see your grandmother?" Mom asked. But I didn't.

I'd spiraled down some psychedelic rabbit hole, and when I first opened my eyes in the hospital room I thought maybe the sheets covering my cold legs were clouds and the nurses hovering over my bed were angels in heaven. I didn't feel in control of my own body. A strange sense of calm washed over me even as the pain squeezed my brain like a clamp. I realized I didn't care what those nurses did to me as long as I didn't hurt anymore afterward. I said a silent prayer that I'd just drift off into a dreamless sleep.

I closed my eyes again. A scene from long ago played on the backs of my eyelids like an old movie reel, the film grainy and choppy. A garden path, the tulips in full bloom and the grass lush and green. My sister, her eyes bright and her cheeks pink, her short hair bouncing as she skipped along the stepping stones. She clutched a large umbrella, and she was singing in the rain. Then just as suddenly as it had appeared, the image was gone.

"I can't save her, John," I whispered, my voice trembling. I tried to sit up, but I didn't have the energy to move. That's when I realized that in my effort to save my sister, I'd been working myself to death.

"We need to take better care of *you*." John's voice sounded far away, though it came from the chair beside my bed. "The doctor said."

The drugs must have started working then because I couldn't feel pain any longer, but I thought I felt tears streaming down my face.

ON THE WAY home from the hospital that night, I promised my husband I'd find better balance at home: I'd limit the long hours on my computer after long days at work, and I'd learn to ask for help with Taylor's Tale when I needed it. But even after that trip to the hospital, I watched my sister lose ground, and though I knew it was unreasonable, I hated myself the times I shut down early, because I worried that I was somehow hurting her chance of survival.

The week before Thanksgiving, I was taking a shower when I got another migraine. I wasn't sure what happened, but I found myself sprawled on a hard, cold surface. I opened my eyes and waited for them to focus on my surroundings: the fine grain of grout; a seagrass basket, stacked high with towels; a glass door cloudy with soap scum. The clothes I'd been wearing that day, strewn in the corner; water droplets and tiny soap bubbles glistening on the tile; a magazine, wrinkled from the steam.

I was wrapped loosely in a damp bath towel, my hair wet and tangled. I realized then that paramedics surrounded me. One of them was taking my pulse. I must have passed out from the migraine.

"Her heart rate is low," he said.

"How low?" John's voice, I realized.

"Unless she's a marathon runner, I'd be concerned."

"She *is* a marathon runner."

"I still think we need to take her in to be safe. Look at her color."

I tried to speak, but my tongue felt heavy and thick and I couldn't form words.

"Here we go." Another voice. I felt hands under my body. They lifted me up. Another set of hands pulled a shirt over my head. I tried to tell the voices this was crazy, that I wasn't sick, that I didn't need to go to the hospital again. Instead I let them carry me out of my house. I remember opening my eyes just long enough to see my neighbors standing in the street, looking on with worried faces, as the medics carried me down the driveway on a gurney and into the back of the waiting ambulance.

"THIS IS HOW it's going to be," John said the next morning, placing a warm mug of coffee in my hands and pulling a chair up next to me at the kitchen table. The words were authoritative, but his tone was gentle. "The ER doctor said these migraines are mostly stress-related. I don't think that's news to either of us."

"No." I studied the antique chestnut table that had once been my mother's. "It's on loan until I have a place for it again one day," she'd said when John loaded it into the back of his truck. But John had refinished it until the beautiful grain of the nineteenth century wood shone, and I knew she'd never ask to have it back.

John put his hand over mine. His knuckles and fingertips were rough from hours of woodworking and playing bass guitar. "Laura," he said, and in my own name I felt the hundreds of experiences we'd shared since meeting our sophomore year of high school, hiking through alpine wildflower meadows and eating ice cream straight from the carton on tables outside the neighborhood Harris Teeter and pushing my sister on the swings as she begged us to go higher, higher, higher. And now I was slipping away, obsessed with fighting the demon killing my sister, so far down the rabbit hole I'd spend three hours battling tech issues with the Taylor's Tale website instead of spending time with my sister who was still alive.

"You feel like if you're not fighting every second of every day, you're selling your sister out," he said softly. "I know you. You can't stand to let Batten win and you can't stand the thought of losing her."

"I can't lose her," I murmured, knowing even as I said the words that it wasn't my choice to make.

"I just don't want you to lose perspective," John said. He took a deep breath. "I know how hard you've worked these past five years. I know you'd do anything to save T and it's one of the reasons why I love you." He ran his finger along the rim of his own coffee mug, which he hadn't touched. "But sometimes you can fight too hard. You can focus on the wrong things. And when you're sick, that's not good for anyone."

I understood before he finished that I had to step back for a while.

"I'm not saying you have to quit," he added, reading my mind. "But we have to get smarter. No more thirty-hour weeks for Taylor's Tale. No more starting new blog posts after midnight when you have to go to work the next day. No more battling IT issues we could pay a webmaster to handle. And Monday, you're calling a neurologist, like the ER doctor said."

I swallowed hard. "Okay."

"I've loved your little sister since the day I followed you home from school and raced you up the stairs to see her for the first time," he said. "I can't lose my sister-in-law and my wife, too."

OF COURSE, MY mother was doing enough for both of us. Even before my hospital visits I'd stepped down as president of Taylor's Tale after two years, and she'd filled the role with vigor that showed her considerable leadership experience, her passion for getting the job done, and a bulldog mentality that we needed to be heard.

"This is *significant* legislation," she said as we walked around the YMCA's indoor track at a fast pace one night. It was mid-January, and sleet pelted the pavement outside. Though I was training for a ten-mile race, I struggled to keep up with my mother. She had never been an athlete, but talking about the disease killing my sister lit a fire within her.

In recent months Mom had developed a near-encyclopedic knowledge of the advocacy issues facing rare disease patients, and with her guidance Taylor's Tale was joining other patient organizations in pushing new legislation known as the ULTRA Act. "The current federal law makes it almost impossible to get new treatments to patients," she went on. "The problem isn't the science—it's the process. We could raise millions of dollars and fix the disease in the lab, but a potential treatment for someone like T could still get stuck in the gauntlet for decades and never go anywhere, all because of regulatory issues. This would streamline the FDA approval process for ultra-rare diseases."

My mother had already been to Washington since taking over as president, attending the first national Conference on Rare Diseases and Orphan Products. She'd gone to large sessions and cornered FDA and NIH people in elevators and bars.

"Did I tell you what one woman from the FDA said to me?" she said.

I couldn't remember. I slowed down and turned toward her, waiting. I couldn't help but think how, even wearing warm-up pants and a t-shirt from Target, she looked like a world beater. "No. What did she say?"

"I asked her to explain why they'd approve a new cancer drug over something to help kids like T," Mom answered. "If she'd played the numbers game I would've understood. Lots of people have cancer; I get it. But do you know what she said?"

I didn't, but I was sure my mother hadn't liked it. "What?"

"She said . . ." Here my mother paused for effect, stepping into the outside lane to dodge a jogger. "'Yes, but *tumors* can *kill* you.' And I wanted to say, 'What the hell do you think Batten disease does?'"

"What *did* you say?"

"That's basically what I said. I just said it politely."

I knew Mom wouldn't forget that woman from the FDA, but she said the real highlight of the conference was the opportunity to hear John Crowley speak in person. Crowley's story was chronicled in *The Cure,* the book she'd bought for members of our original steering committee years earlier, right after Taylor's diagnosis. I thought of my mother's fighting words the afternoon she distributed those books and decided she hadn't changed much, even though she had a few new scars.

"HAS YOUR MOTHER told you what the kids at Fletcher are doing?" Dad said. "The teachers are helping, but I think it's mostly the kids." We were watching a basketball game at my parents' house, part of my effort to find balance in light of the pact I'd made with John. I hadn't done any Taylor's Tale work in several days, and I'd been pleasantly surprised to find that the sky hadn't come crashing down on me and the fight against Batten disease hadn't suddenly come to a screeching halt.

"She hasn't." I peered into the kitchen, where my mother was engrossed in a scientific abstract on her laptop and Taylor was working with soft modeling clay to keep her hands strong. "What's going on?"

"Some fundraiser. You'll have to ask her." My father would lie down on railroad tracks for any of his children, but it wasn't his nature to be involved in Taylor's Tale. He was more extroverted than my mother and found himself squarely in his element at cocktail parties and dinners, events Mom hated, but he left the business side of our fight against Batten disease to my mother and me. Even my brother Stephen had joined the board the previous year, but my father, who'd sold life insurance my whole life, liked to say he didn't have any useful skills to give to the cause. Obviously that was just an excuse. I think being Taylor's dad was painful enough for him, and he didn't want any more of Batten disease in his life than was necessary. Lately, I understood.

"What fundraiser are they doing at Fletcher?" I asked Mom, walking into the kitchen.

"Some cardio craze thing with Andre Hairston," Mom said, not looking up from her computer screen. "Do you remember Andre?"

"Of course." Andre was a local celebrity and fitness instructor who taught classes at our YMCA and had a magnetic personality. Everyone knew Andre.

"I don't have any details. I just know the kids and staff asked Andre to lead a session in the school gym, and they're raising money for us. I'll check my calendar and send the date to you." She saved the document she was working on and glanced at my sister, who'd stayed quiet. I knew that often meant she was hanging on every word. I wondered what she must think about the business side of our fight against Batten disease—supporting the mission of Taylor's Tale. I wished I could ask her how she felt, but that would mean we'd also have to talk about the disease that was killing her. Mostly I wished we didn't have a charity, because that would mean my sister didn't have Batten disease.

"Taylor? It's time to go to bed." Mom pried the clay from my sister's fingers and helped her stand.

I DIDN'T HEAR anything else about the fundraiser for a few weeks. Then when the big day arrived in mid-February, my father called me not long after he dropped Taylor off at school.

"Half the kids on campus were wearing purple or pink," he said, his voice cracking.

I ran out of my office after lunch and drove seven miles to The Fletcher School. My mind was racing, and once the driver behind me had to tap on his horn when my attention wandered at a traffic light. After I'd pulled into a space on the campus and turned off the car, I took a moment to close my eyes and refocus.

When I entered the gym, I walked into a sea of glitter, sparkle, and love. I got a funny catch in my throat as I took it all in. There were so many people I couldn't see the floor.

Teachers were wearing tutus and tie-dye shirts, and the girls were wearing feathery boas and pink tights and strings of beads and dangly earrings that swayed as they danced. Even the boys were covered in pink body paint, as if they were at a powder puff football game. Some of them were wearing tutus, too. A lot of the kids wore homemade t-shirts with phrases like "Tay Tay you rock" and "we love you" and "4 Taylor's Tale."

I won't forget the stories I heard from teachers in the gym that day. The kids had to pay five dollars to attend the event. But one student donated the contents of his allowance jar—more than one hundred and fifty dollars. A girl in the upper school had paid her five dollars, but the day before the event, she told her teacher she wanted her money back. When asked why, she produced a twenty dollar bill. "I got the money for my birthday," she told the teacher. "I saw on the website that a lot of kids with Batten disease don't get to celebrate their sixteenth birthday, so I think Taylor's Tale should have my birthday money." Some kids turned fundraising into a friendly competition. "I found three dollars in my jacket yesterday," one middle school student told his friends in the cafeteria. "I'm giving it to Taylor's Tale. How much are you donating?" My sister's friend Charlotte told me boys who'd never participated at school dances were the ones leading the crowd in the front of the gym; other boys had fought over her tutus and texted the girls requests for custom-made t-shirts the day before the event.

But it was watching my sister, dressed in a purple boa and purple necklace and a t-shirt her friends had decorated, that made me blink back tears. Flanked by the other girls, she danced throughout the entire event. Several times Andre jumped into step with her and chanted her name, and she'd clap and laugh and jump up and down like she was on an invisible pogo stick. Boys I didn't recognize asked her to dance with them. When Andre and the crowd turned to face a different wall, they had a gentle way of making sure Taylor rotated, too. When Andre invited Taylor and her friends onstage toward the end of the program, the other girls helped my sister navigate the stairs so she wouldn't get left behind.

The students raised thirty-five hundred dollars that day—support for a future project to save future Taylors. I tried not to think about money or time, though. It felt better to focus on the heart those kids put into the event and the kindness they showed toward my sister.

Watching Taylor's friends guide her on to the stage, I saw, in a single instant, the depth of my sister's courage and the reality that her path and the paths of her peers had diverged. They'd be learning to drive in a year; before long they'd be visiting colleges. Meanwhile, my sister was sliding backward. Batten was gaining speed. Though I didn't know it then, the cardio craze fundraiser was the last big event Taylor would attend at The Fletcher School.

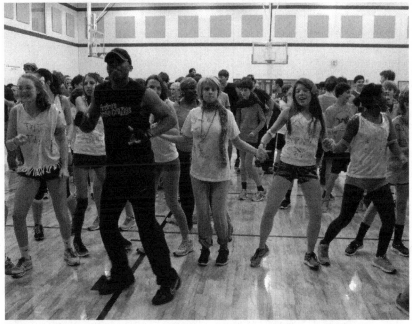

Taylor's Fletcher School classmates turn their gym into a sea of sparkle, glitter, and love, 2012

Chapter 17

EARLY THAT SPRING, my mother flew overnight to gray London for the international congress on Batten disease.

"They rerouted us through Washington," she said in an email that arrived early the next morning. "I did my best sardine imitation in economy class. No time to sleep—the first session is in an hour. Will write more later."

At my urging, Mom had agreed to keep a journal for a daily "Notes from London" series on the Taylor's Tale blog. The summaries arrived in my inbox each night as late as three a.m. London time. She said the campus of the University of London's Royal Holloway College looked like something out of *Harry Potter*, yet the college's conference venue was modern and sleek. She didn't like the food—"This is a college, so the portions are gigantic and I've not suffered for lack of carbs." I imagined my health-conscious mother facing a plate of fish and chips and wished I could FedEx a salad.

The morning my mother arrived, she'd stumbled upon the initial organizing meeting of the Batten Disease International Alliance. Though she hadn't been aware of the meeting, the woman at the registration table had urged her to attend. "She said she knows Taylor's Tale and we should be involved," Mom said in her first email. "I guess I'll go." My mother had always been a bit of a lone wolf, but she'd isolated herself more recently. I could tell that more and more, she just wanted to put her head down and get things done on her own.

"Steve Gray is here, too, along with the usual suspects," she said after the second day. "Also, two scientists with a company called BioMarin. They're working on late infantile Batten." I couldn't help but think about how detached my mother sounded in these early emails. I kept hoping she'd say something about how the conference made her feel or if she thought the trip to Europe had been worthwhile. I wondered if I'd been expecting too much by asking her to keep a journal or if she was still jetlagged from her flight.

On the third morning, my mother ran up the hill from her dorm to the main building to get a good seat for the session on novel therapies.

"The team working on enzyme replacement therapy for late infantile Batten is close to a clinical trial," she wrote late that night. "They showed videos of the long-haired dachshunds in the canine study. The dogs were in the end-stages of the disease and very sick. They suffered from symptoms like blindness and persistent myoclonic jerks—involuntary muscle twitches I've seen in T, too. A lot of people turned away from the screen. I wanted to grab their shoulders and make them watch. 'This isn't Hollywood,' I wanted to say. 'This is what happens to children with this disease. If it breaks your heart to see it in an animal, what are you going to do about it to save a child?'"

THREE DAYS AFTER Mom returned from London, I met my family for dinner at a deli down the street. My mother still looked as if she hadn't recovered from her transatlantic trip, and I remember thinking how she seemed to be trying harder than usual to be cheerful.

We ate our sandwiches and soup, and Taylor ate her macaroni and cheese, and we sat and talked for a while. At first glance, my sister—now thirteen—looked the part of a teenager in her cheerleader shorts and pink headband. Her hair was cut in a cute bob, a style that worked well with the dark, thick hair that had come after the stem cell transplant. Mom once said, "If you want great hair, just shave it off."

Taylor ate quietly, listening to our chatter. I tried not to notice that she was eating her macaroni with her fingers because she was losing her motor skills and couldn't hold a fork any longer. I thought about how, if things were normal, she'd be telling me about her day at school. But Taylor didn't talk much anymore. Her processing skills had suffered so much that it was difficult for her to keep up in a conversation, and when she did speak, she often repeated the same phrase until it drove us crazy. After she saw *Pirates of the Caribbean* for the first time, she started saying, "I like Jack . . . and Jack . . . and Jack . . . and Jack . . . and Jack . . ." in reference to the main character until we all hated the movie. I didn't understand then that before long, I'd give anything to hear Taylor say, "I like Jack."

After the tables around us had emptied, Stephen mentioned the time. We stood to leave; my mother took my sister's arm and pulled her to her feet. It hurt to watch because it showed a lot of what my sister had lost in a single snapshot—her vision, her spatial awareness, and her ability to process the situation and understand it was time to stand up and walk toward the door.

"I want to hear more about London this weekend," I said to Mom in the parking lot, our shadows lengthening on the pavement as the last of the daylight faded beyond the trees. "Oh, and did you get that email I forwarded from our website? From the dad in New Zealand whose son was just diagnosed? Something about new drug targets and labs in Europe—it was long and I only scanned it."

Suddenly my mother's face hardened, though she didn't seem angry at me. "Jim, help Taylor get in the car," she said over her shoulder, motioning for Dad to take my sister's arm. She turned back to me. "Yes, I saw the email. And do you know how I really want to respond?"

I didn't say anything, shaken by the tone in her voice, like she was ready for a fight. Instinctively, I looked around to see if my sister could hear. She was strapped into the front seat of my parents' car parked next to mine; the doors were closed. I turned back to my mother, who was just warming up.

"I want to say, You're not going to find a magic bullet or a medicine man in your Google searches. Get out there and help us raise money for a real treatment with some of that time you're searching on the computer. Parents are so desperate—looking for anything. How well I understand them." Now she stole a glance at my sister, and in the fluorescent glow of the parking lot lights, I saw that my mother was crying.

"You know, Mark Sands said a telling thing to me at that workshop in Bethesda," she went on. "We were sitting in the lobby of the Marriott. I can still see the sofa and the people milling around us. It's like a photograph imprinted on my brain—that point in my life where I finally understood and woke up to our certain future for Taylor. Mark said he dreads meeting the new families at Batten Association conferences. They come into the lobby full of hope and desire to find the answer for *their* child. They believe it *can* and *will* be in time if they put together enough bake sales and 5K runs. What he said that stuck with me is that each and every child far enough along in the disease process to make it to a family conference has no hope of ever benefiting from a treatment. If they're at a conference, they have a diagnosis, meaning they're already too far progressed."

I leaned against my own car, suddenly worried I'd lose my balance. My legs felt like rubber, and my voice was caught in my throat. Usually I had a response ready. In private I was angry, sad, exhausted—but around my mother I tried to be a rock for her. Now I had nothing to say. Even though I'd been thinking the same thing for months, hearing it out loud made it real, and I was more scared than I'd ever been.

"That was the moment I knew I could quit," my mother continued, lowering her voice. "No way could I help T. We were too far in and she was too far gone. Yes, I could quit. Or—I could keep fighting like hell and kick Batten's butt."

"You're not a quitter," I whispered, a desperate attempt to fill the charged air between us.

"I detest people who give up, people who quit, people who sit back and wait for someone else to make things better, then take advantage of the contribution. Everyone can't be expected to approach life in the same way. But if we quit, who'll take out this monster? We need *every last human* who hates Batten to suit up and help. I want to say to that father in New Zealand, get off the Internet looking for someone else to change your life. For God's sake, *help*."

I had a sick feeling in the pit of my stomach. I knew I hadn't been fighting as hard since my second trip to the emergency room. I knew I'd gotten doctor's orders to reduce my load, and I knew Mom wanted me to be healthy. But still, I hated myself for not being invincible for her, and for Taylor.

My heart pounding, I threw my arms around my mother, closing the space that separated us. I'd half expected to see a crowd of people gawking at us after that emotional speech. But even Dad had taken Taylor home, and my brother's truck was gone, and the black night and emptiness were all around us.

IT WAS EARLY May, with the end of school only three weeks away, flower beds bursting with color, and the sky on clear days an impossible shade of blue. All of us were traveling to Folly Beach that weekend for the wedding of our friend Callie to her college sweetheart, Will. We stayed right on the ocean in a house called My Blue Heaven; it had a large deck and steps that went right down to the sand. The boys drank Coronas with lime slices, and Taylor sat in a sliver of shade with a bucket of plastic beads. Beneath the brim of her pink straw hat my sister's eyes were slack, because they couldn't focus on anything. Her gaze was just *off*, an effect of Batten disease that had become more pronounced that year. I put an arm around her and closed my eyes, stretching my legs in the sunshine baking the gray cedar boards of the deck floor. As I drifted off to sleep, I thought staying right there would make me just as happy as going to a wedding.

Eventually I did peel myself out of my chair, though, and my mother washed and combed and blow-dried my sister's hair. It was thick and wavy, and when it caught the sunlight just right, it looked like pure honey. Taylor wore strappy sandals that showed off her pedicure and a sundress the color of a juicy tangerine that made her look grown up. For a moment I convinced myself she didn't have Batten disease; however, it was difficult getting her down the windy staircase of our beach house and across the soft sand to one of the chairs reserved for elderly grandparents and others unable to stand for the ceremony by the sea. *She needs a wheelchair,* I said to myself. *Maybe not all the time,* I thought quickly. *Just for times like this.*

But when we filed into the bride's house with all of the guests for the reception, Taylor immediately took my hand and pulled me toward the sound of the music. "Let's dance," she said in a childish, happy voice. I couldn't help but notice the irony—the girl who'd just minutes earlier sat in a chair because she couldn't stand, dragging me onto a dance floor. I followed her to the middle of the room and twirled her around, even though nobody else was dancing.

Long after dinner, my sister was still dancing. Maybe it was from baking in the sun earlier, but I was exhausted. "Why don't you take another turn with Taylor?" I said to my father, who'd floated in and out of our dance circle to mingle with other guests.

"Okay," he said, setting his half-full beer on our table and taking my sister's hands. "Come on, T." He led her onto the makeshift dance floor, which by now was empty again. Somewhere behind me, Callie hugged friends goodnight, and I pictured her father-daughter dance earlier that evening and my own dance with my father at my wedding six years before, and my cheeks burned with anger, because I knew deep down Taylor and Dad would never have that chance. A lamp in the corner cast a golden glow into the room against a backdrop of darkening sky. And as I watched my sister dance with my dad, I pushed her struggles out of my mind, and I thought about how her light, too, burned brightly, in spite of the monster. That was the last time I saw my sister really break free from Batten disease.

MY SISTER'S LAST day at Fletcher fell on the first day of June. It was a beautiful day, more suited to a beginning than an end.

I knew my parents had suffered for weeks over their choice, but eventually, they took the only feasible road. They were sending her to a public school that had a special, self-contained class for students with significant disabilities. Because Fletcher was a private school and Taylor its only blind student, my parents had paid out-of-pocket for her specialized, one-on-one instruction with a vision teacher. But it was Batten disease, more than money, that stopped my parents from sending Taylor back to Fletcher for ninth grade; they would have sold their house to keep her in the best situation. "She's just not learning anymore," Mom conceded to me one night, her eyes filling with tears. "If we thought she was still getting something out of it—"

"You don't have to explain to me," I said, stopping her. "I get it." In my heart I wanted them to take the money they'd save on Fletcher and travel with Taylor. She'd always wanted to go to Hawaii, and my parents could use the time away from home, too. But inside I knew my sister would never make it to Hawaii. Just going to the North Carolina mountains was becoming more difficult; how could she possibly endure a twelve-hour travel day to get to the islands?

I remembered Taylor's fifth grade graduation ceremony, three years earlier; Fletcher had called it Moving Up Day. Taylor had won awards for her "inspirational attitude" and her "amazing accomplishment of learning braille." Now the Perkins Brailler she'd once been so proud of was gathering dust in my mother's basement office, and the milestone of finishing eighth grade felt more like moving out than moving up.

I made it to the school just in time for the ceremony that afternoon. Afterward I met Taylor in the lobby, where she stood next to one of her teachers, clutching a certificate.

"I finished," she said bashfully.

"You finished," I whispered, both proud and heartbroken as I scooped her up in a hug.

PLACE AND TIME had always connected us to Chris and Wendy Hawkins, who lived near our hometown and whose sons, Brandon and Jeremy, were both diagnosed around the same time as Taylor. But we rarely saw the Hawkins family; while we got along fine, we shied away from what we felt would have been friendships predicated on a shared tragedy. Most Batten families only knew my mother and me, and some people thought we were aloof because we skipped all of the social gatherings at family conferences, though in reality we just treated the meetings like business trips and didn't know how to clock out. But each spring I saw the Hawkins family at a 5K fundraiser Chris organized, so in a way I'd still watched the boys grow up. Brandon had always been tall like his dad, and this year he towered over me at six feet, two inches. Jeremy had been diagnosed early because of his older brother; when I met him five years earlier he'd been a bright-eyed, chatty ball of energy and mostly pre-symptomatic, but now he stumbled over his words and walked with a cane. The decline was all too familiar.

The first weekend in June, a runner friend of the Hawkins' named Jeff McGonnell was circling the town green in Davidson, a lakeside college town just north of Charlotte, for twenty-four hours to raise money for the Batten Association. I signed up to run with Jeff for an hour; John was out of town for work, and I drove to Davidson solo after lunch.

Walking toward the green from my parking spot on Main Street, I saw a band of sweaty, singlet-clad runners following Jeff around the quarter-mile perimeter of the shaded square and the tent Chris had set up with the Batten Association banner. The blue sky, the green grass, and the charm of the college town's Soda Shop and sidewalk cafes made me feel as if I was a million miles from home and nothing could touch me, even though Brandon and Jeremy and the specter of Batten disease sat in lawn chairs fifty feet away. I felt an unexpected jolt of happiness, like the sensation I got in college whenever I turned in my last exam of the semester. I quickened my pace and smiled at families holding ice cream cones and shopping bags as we passed on the sidewalk.

The moment I reached the Hawkins family, I understood it wasn't the pretty day or the quaint college town that had made me so cheerful. For the first time, it felt good to be in a place where someone else understood what I was living, because they were living it, too. Where I didn't have to describe the terrible things or even say anything at all, because they already knew. I took an awful sort of comfort in knowing we weren't the only ones who'd seen and felt and touched this kind of pain.

I'd run a 10K by the time my parents arrived with Taylor, parking in one of the handicap spots right behind Chris's tent. I had run for an hour like I'd promised, but I couldn't stop. Maybe I was afraid to get back in my car and drive home to Charlotte, but running had never felt so good. I ran laps in musty wigs and flowered hats, ragged grass skirts and hot boxing gloves for extra dollars for the Batten Association. Each time I circled the green, I stole a glance at my sister in one of the chairs under the tent, her head slumped and her eyes sluggish from the warmth of the June day. I saw her vacant look, and anger crept in to mix with the joy. My father bought me two oatmeal raisin cookies from The Soda Shop, and I ran another seven miles. I completed a half marathon just as Jeff started his final lap.

I didn't feel tired driving home later, even though I'd run around a quarter-mile patch of grass in crazy costumes for most of a warm afternoon. I felt alive, renewed, and ready for battle. I'd started this race to beat Batten disease, and I wanted to finish it. Sometimes it hurt, but not so much that I needed to stop. I'd come so far already. I figured I might as well keep running.

WE WENT TO Mom and Dad's for the Fourth of July. During dessert, my father mentioned he'd driven the ten miles to South Carolina for cheap gas and bought fireworks. I thought of summers at Grandma Kathryn and Papa Jerry's beach house on North Carolina's Oak Island, celebrating the Fourth across the canal in Southport's waterfront park. I could almost smell our picnics of buttery biscuits and crispy fried chicken and sweet tea on a scratchy blanket under a hazy blue sky. We watched boats drift by and filled our bellies and told stories. Stephen and I liked to pick our way through the other quilts to the pier to buy snow cones and glow-necklaces before the sun sank beneath the horizon. When the last rays of sunlight faded to darkness, the fireworks lit up the night.

It'd been fifteen years since I last saw the Cape Fear River sky bursting with sparkling streaks of color. I looked around my parents' kitchen and realized how much our world had changed since those summers at Oak Island. My grandmother's Lewy body dementia had gotten so bad, Papa Jerry hadn't taken Mom's invitation to spend the holiday in Charlotte this year. I thought about how my sister hadn't even been born when my grandfather sold the beach house.

My mother had baked macaroni, and the kitchen was still warm from the oven, but suddenly I had chills.

"I think we all need some fireworks," I said to my father. I pushed my chair back from the table and helped Taylor stand.

In the driveway minutes later, my sister sat in a golf chair between Mom and me, listening to the striking of matches and the scrambling that followed as Stephen and John helped my father light the fireworks. Taylor squealed each time they shot a Roman candle or bottle rocket into the black night. As the fireworks exploded over the front yard, I called out the colors, one by one, to my blind sister. I held her hand, and I watched the dying of the light.

Chapter 18

I'LL NEVER FORGET my first day of ninth grade. I'd gone to a magnet elementary school for seven years, and after sixth grade my friends scattered to middle schools all over town. The dividing line for two rival high schools was in our neighborhood, and all of my middle school friends lived in the other district, so two years later I faced another round of goodbyes.

My father drove me to the big high school that first morning. Classes started early, and dew still glistened on the fresh-cut grass fringing the traffic circle. I had braces and freckles on my nose from soccer camp, and as I got ready to step out of the car, I clutched the straps of my backpack against my chest so the other kids couldn't see that my hands were shaking.

"You'll do just fine, sweetie," Dad said, leaning across the armrest to give me a hug. I glanced over my shoulder at the kids clustered around the flagpole and wriggled out of his grasp.

"Love you, Dad," I said, opening the car door and taking a deep breath.

When the bell rang at the end of my science class, I sat glued to my seat, my limbs frozen; lunch came next, and the cafeteria, teeming with kids who all seemed to have found a crowd three hours into the new school year, terrified me. I peeled myself out of my chair only after I noticed the teacher peering at me over a stack of books and papers in her arm as she shuffled toward the door, looking for a free hand to turn out the light.

I'll never forget the roller coaster sensation that roiled my insides as I walked into the crowded cafeteria and found my way to the pizza line, just as I'll never forget the popular-looking girl who invited me to sit at her table. That moment ensured my survival of ninth grade. I made the soccer team, enjoyed my classes, found niches in journalism and art, and made a lot of friends. I never ate lunch with that girl again, but I always remembered what she did for me.

On Taylor's first day at her new school, Mom sent a photo of my sister standing in my parents' driveway as they were getting ready to leave. She was wearing skinny jeans and a striped top with strappy sandals, and my mother had blow-dried her hair. She was tall and slender and seemed like she'd been cut out of an ad for teen fashion, except that she'd forgotten to look at the camera and her posture was stilted—the result of muscular atrophy and problems with balance.

"She looks beautiful," I replied. But my fingers shook when I typed the words. I knew my sister wouldn't go to class every day, because she couldn't handle a full schedule. I knew she couldn't write for the school paper or join any clubs or try out for the soccer team. I knew she wouldn't see even the smiles of the people who'd be there to help her experience something normal like high school, at least in some small way. I knew she might not have four years.

THROUGH THE SUMMER and into the fall, my mother had been following Steve Gray's work on the ultra-rare childhood disease GAN at the University of North Carolina. Despite my Uncle David's initial skepticism, she hadn't given up hope. In September she ordered copies of a book about gene therapy called *The Forever Fix* and distributed them to the Taylor's Tale board as assigned reading. "Pay close attention to the chapters on a little girl named Hannah and her family," Mom said in an email to everyone. "They're funding Steve Gray's work at UNC—something we should consider doing for Batten." The last time my mother had placed a bulk order for books had led to the founding of Taylor's Tale. I wondered where this one would lead.

The energy I'd felt at the end of my unexpected half marathon on Davidson's town green in June kept me going even as the nights grew cooler and the leaves began to change. I felt encouraged about where we were headed. In October, Mom invited Hannah's mother, Lori Sames, to travel to Charlotte from her home near Albany, New York, to talk about the GAN research at our fall board meeting.

Lori had large hazel eyes and wore her long hair pulled back loosely in a large clip. When she strode into the conference room wheeling a suitcase, it was easy to imagine she rode horses and spoke in a smooth, slow lilt, like water lapping against a shore. But Lori talked in rapid bursts riddled with complex jargon, reeling off phrases like "GLP toxicology studies" and "Adeno Associated Virus serotype 9" and "recombinant DNA." She spoke passionately about the research Hannah's Hope had funded and the progress they'd made, but her language was so technical that it was difficult for the fundraising and marketing pros and accountants on our board to follow her. I scribbled notes on a pad until my wrist ached.

"I'm exhausted," Mom said when she called me much later, after she'd taken Lori out for coffee on the way to her hotel. "And here I thought *I* was dedicated. It's no wonder Lori's accomplished so much. She never rests."

"So what do you think about the GAN project now?" I asked, because that's all I really cared about. "What are our next steps?"

"We're funding gene therapy for Batten. It's the only way."

STEVE GRAY NEEDED more money to study infantile Batten disease than Taylor's Tale had in the bank, so after Lori left Mom went to work finding partners to help us fund the infantile Batten part of a proposed parallel study on infantile and late infantile Batten disease at the UNC Gene Therapy Center. She had them before Thanksgiving, like I'd known she would. "We'll be one of six funders for the two forms combined," she told me while we were reviewing the holiday menu, determining who'd cook the turkey and stuffing and spiral ham. "The money will cover the work for two years. In the meantime, we can watch the GAN research evolve—maybe even make it to clinical trial. That's our goal, too."

"I believe in Steve Gray, and I believe in Taylor's Tale," I said. "We'll get there." I didn't know Steve, who'd been in our home state all this time, as well as I knew most of the multinational scientists who were regulars at the Batten Association conferences. But I'd follow my mother's intuition to the ends of the earth, and after watching my sister decline that year, I felt like it was time to take a leap of faith.

As the details unfolded in the days that followed, I learned that *all* of the funders were charities founded by families losing a child to Batten disease. Charities with devastated parents at the helm, and no paid staff. *Is this the best the world can do for children like Taylor?* I wondered.

With so many players involved, the deliberations dragged. "We'll have our project," Mom assured me. I was in awe of my mother that fall. She'd become an expert on the disease killing my sister and a fierce advocate for three hundred fifty million people suffering from a rare disorder. She asked tough questions when everyone else was too afraid or too busy, and she demanded the best out of anyone with a chance in hell of giving kids like Taylor a rosier future. I'd served as president of Taylor's Tale for two years, and I knew I'd never stop telling our story. But watching her in those days as the orange and gold and crimson leaves fell to the ground, foreshadowing yet another season, I knew she was and would always be our leader.

In the meantime, I ran. My third half marathon was in late November, and I hadn't trained so much as I'd maintained my waistline during the summer and early autumn. One Saturday I went for my first long run in weeks, skipping through leaves on a sidewalk lined with tall oaks. I remembered a day not so long ago, when Taylor, her long hair streaming behind her, jumped into Dad's piles of leaves with unrestrained bliss. A day in another lifetime. I thought about how, as the seasons changed, they brought new unknowns for my sister and our family.

There'd been a storm the previous week, and the branches of some of the oaks were almost bare. In the spring, they would be reborn, their canopies bursting with color. As I exited the tunnel of trees, blinking in the suddenly bright sunlight, I thought about how my blind sister would never see the seasons change again.

THE MORNING OF my half marathon, I caught the light rail uptown with my friend Kelli. Kelli's husband Danny was recording an album with John in the North Carolina mountains, so Kelli had spent the night with me in Charlotte and was running for Taylor, too.

Earlier that week I'd received a message on my blog from the father of a student at The Fletcher School. He and his son Nicholas, who was a year behind my sister and had just started the eighth grade at Fletcher, were running the half marathon. "Neither of us are runners but we are doing it for the challenge," he wrote. "I mentioned to Nicholas that Taylor did a 5K without stopping and I told him we can't even think about walking or slowing down before mile three because no matter

how 'tired' we may be, we need to push through just like Taylor did."
I felt inspired because others still honored my sister, but I also felt sad
because, as her peers grew older, they were unintentionally leaving her
behind.

Though I'd started to see myself as an experienced runner, I couldn't
stop thinking about how little I'd trained for this race. "I'm just going to
have fun today," I said to Kelli as we speed-walked toward the start line
against a bitter wind. The words were more for myself than my friend.
"No time goal."

When the gun sounded, we inched forward with the others, two
specks of purple in a throng of thousands. We walked till the pack
leaders burst ahead, making room for everyone else. After what felt like
an eternity, we broke free. I said goodbye to my friend and shot ahead,
settling into my own pace.

I knew right away that things would go better than expected. The air
didn't feel nearly as cold as it had just moments earlier when we'd jogged
in place to stay warm, and it felt good when it filled my lungs. Each time
I approached a hill, I found an unexpected burst of energy. My head felt
clear. I was on pace for a personal record.

But after a long climb around mile five, I got winded. I thought
about slowing down until I remembered how Taylor had run part of the
same course in her first 5K and never once stopped to walk, even when
she fell and scraped her knees. I thought about Nicholas and his dad
and my friend Kelli, somewhere on the course running for Taylor, and
I didn't stop.

Less than a mile from the finish line, I ran beneath the bridge where,
two years earlier, I'd seen the blind man running with a cane. This time
I was alone under the bridge, but I could see the image of the blind half
marathon runner perfectly in my mind, and it made me think of my
little sister, fighting a demon of a disease at home.

As the end of the course came into view, I tweaked my left leg.
The pain felt so excruciating that I thought I'd torn a muscle. I'd never
envisioned crawling across the finish line and didn't like even the
thought. I wanted to sprint, but I was limping.

Was this what it was coming down to in the end? I'd given it my best,
but my body had hit its limit. In my heart I knew I couldn't run Batten
disease out of Taylor's life. I knew I couldn't chase down a cure, no matter

how fast I ran. I knew the running was for me. But in that moment, I hated that my best wasn't good enough. I forgot I was running a race. I hated that our world was falling away beneath us and everything we'd ever known and taken for granted was slipping out of our grasps and my sister was still going to die.

But our fight against Batten disease wasn't a sprint. It was a marathon. And the best distance runners succeed by reserving energy so they'll be fresh when they have to climb the toughest hills. Elite marathoners know better than to expend all their energy in the first few miles of the race. I had to face Batten disease one day at a time. I'd shaped myself into a distance runner by approaching a long race in small chunks. It was easier to think about running a great two miles—the distance between aid stations. After my hospital scares, I'd finally started to understand that taking care of myself was just as important as hard work; otherwise, I'd crash and burn before I reached my goal. Similar to stringing together a bunch of strong miles, I needed to string together a bunch of good days.

My sudden injury made me angry and Batten disease made me angry, but as more able-bodied runners passed me en route to the finish line, it dawned on me that there was only so much we could do to win the race at hand. It was a tragic situation, and nothing that happened in my life—no matter how wonderful it might be—could ever replace what we'd lost and stood to lose. But a fast runner with a bum leg wasn't any good to anyone, just like I wasn't good to anyone when I was in my darkest place. I couldn't help my sister if I based my survival on my chance of ensuring hers.

Somehow, I managed to jog-hop the last one hundred yards of Thunder Road's 13.1-mile course. When I looked over my shoulder at the running clock suspended above the timing mats, I discovered I'd set a new personal record. As I wrapped myself in an aluminum blanket and poured water down my throat, I found that the pain in my leg was gone.

ON CHRISTMAS MORNING, John and I drove to Greensboro with my family to say goodbye to my Grandma Kathryn. My grandparents' small house in the retirement community near Uncle David and Aunt Holly was cold and dimly lit and didn't feel like a home. My grandparents' house in Raleigh had always made me happy; the smells of strong brewed coffee and fresh-baked pound cakes wafted from the kitchen; family photos and favorite poems covered the walls, and my grandmother's soothing voice warmed the room. Since her illness had advanced, Papa's model ships and chipped figurines and dog-eared magazines he had bought at yard sales and flea markets had come to clutter every surface of her now dusty, once lovingly polished heirloom furniture.

My grandmother looked like a ghost lying in the hospital bed that had been wheeled into the sitting room. Listening to her breathe, I wished I'd come earlier. But the grandmother who'd taught me to find the best seashells on the North Carolina shore and taken care of me when I was most vulnerable and made us promise to fight for Taylor's life till the end, had been gone for a long time already. I watched her thin chest rise and fall beneath the white sheet and wished I had an explanation for everything. But terrible things had happened to my family and I couldn't find any meaning in them at all.

Once, several months before, a friend asked me if I believe in God. I believed, I said, but I was angry with Him for a long time. I had to search my soul after Taylor's diagnosis. I struggled with the concept of a world that includes Batten disease.

It didn't happen overnight, but somewhere along the way—I don't quite remember when—I had made my peace with God. I came to the realization that God doesn't inflict pain and suffering; rather, He gives us strength to overcome it. But if we want to survive, we have to believe.

Isn't that all any of us can do—endure life's darkest turns and accept that we might not find a light around the bend? Wouldn't my grandmother and Taylor be willing to meet God halfway? If they were able, wouldn't they keep marching onward in their search for the light?

My family was all around me then. My uncle said a prayer, then placed two fingers on my grandmother's wrist, held them there, and shook his head. My mother wept. But I couldn't cry. My eyes were frozen knots of tears, and my body was still as ice.

Chapter 19

THE DAY WE buried my grandmother was gray and still and cold. John and I gave eulogies at the memorial service in the Raleigh church where she'd sung in the choir and my parents had been married. My husband looked tall and strong in his charcoal suit, but he cried softly behind me on the church lectern as I shared happy stories about how Grandma Kathryn and I wrote poetry together and made our famous secret recipe toast and watched ships drift down the Cape Fear River. A knot formed in my throat when I talked about the difficult final years she had endured. I hated brain disease for stealing the people I loved. I hated not being able to say a proper goodbye.

My mother struggled, too; she was the last one to leave the casket following the graveside service. I watched as she ran her hand up and down the polished wood. Before she walked away, she took a single rose.

WHEN THE DUST settled after my grandmother's death, I lost myself in work. The healthcare system I worked for was going through a major rebranding, and as part of the marketing team, I was under enormous pressure to write copy for websites and print materials and organize employee events before the spring deadline. In the meantime, my mother had worked her magic on the research front; by mid-January Taylor's Tale was preparing to announce that we were signing on to co-fund Steve Gray's gene therapy project for Batten disease at UNC.

Due to an agreement with our co-funders, we were compelled to keep the details of the new project confidential until the official announcement on World Rare Disease Day at the end of February. But I wanted to build interest in advance of the breakfast event we were planning to announce the news, so one night, I posted a short message on social media promising that Taylor's Tale would have an exciting update about the fight against Batten disease to share in the coming weeks.

The post struck a nerve with one parent who had already lost a child to Batten disease. She asked why we couldn't just share the news *now*? When I explained that we weren't able to provide additional details yet, she lashed out at Taylor's Tale. How could we be so cruel as to tease desperate parents, only to make them wait? She pulled other families into the fray. Her posts turned belligerent. She accused us of lying. We didn't have real news, she said. I took the conversation offline, but she continued to post defamatory comments on the Taylor's Tale page until I finally blocked her access.

It was one of the most perplexing experiences I'd had since my sister's diagnosis, and in some ways it was one of the hardest. I wanted to tell that mother, *None of us asked for this. Nothing about it is easy. I'm hurting just like you. My sister is going to die just like your son died. I'm doing the best I can to beat this disease, because I hate it as much as you do. If my best isn't good enough, I'm really sorry, but miracles don't happen overnight, or even in a few years.*

TO SETTLE DOWN after the social media disaster, I focused my attention on our announcement. My mom had decided that she needed to be in Washington the week of Rare Disease Day, which meant she'd miss our breakfast announcement. "Taylor's Tale should be there— attending events on Capitol Hill, learning, and making connections," she said on a Sunday afternoon in early February while we were walking our dogs in her neighborhood. Her breath was visible in the frigid, damp air. "Knocking on doors in the halls of Congress. Sharing our story with everyone from senators to legislative assistants. Lobbying for improved access to treatments for people like T." She pulled my sister's dog, Sunny, out of the pine needles she'd been exploring in their neighbor's yard and turned to look at me.

"I wish your grandmother had lived to see this day," she said.

"I do, too," I said. "She would be so proud."

"You know, Taylor's Tale wouldn't have happened without her." She looked around, as if she expected Grandma Kathryn to step out from behind the tall oaks standing watch over the quiet street. "Those first few weeks after the diagnosis, I cried all the time. One day we were talking on the phone, and suddenly she told me I had to come home to Raleigh.

I didn't want to make the trip, but she insisted. When I got to her house she dragged out a weeks-old, dog-eared copy of a magazine article about the Crowleys and their fight against Pompe disease. The reporter had interviewed a doctor at Duke. 'You can do this,' she said. 'This family did it and they're working with people right here in North Carolina.' Then she dragged me to the bookstore and bought two copies of *The Cure* and made me promise I'd read the book. I said I'd think about it. I told her nobody in North Carolina knew anything about Batten disease. She was mad at me the whole way home. 'You're giving up before you even start,' she said."

"But you read the book," I said, a smile playing on my lips.

"I did. Then I ordered a whole case. And—well, you know the rest."

"Now she's an angel, watching down on us." My heart fluttered as I realized the full meaning of the story my mother had shared. "And she was right," I said slowly. "Our answer was here in North Carolina all along. His name is Steve Gray."

"It hurts that I can't be in town this week to share our big news, but I'm not worried," Mom said, her eyes watering. "I'm leaving Taylor's Tale in good hands."

"Thanks, Mom." I kicked at a pebble in the street and watched it skip into the grass. "I'm glad Steve is coming to talk about the project." I'd been working on my talk for the breakfast, but I hadn't made much progress. Normally words came easily to me, but I wanted this to be perfect. The pressure was high. I sensed that we were on the cusp of something great, and I wanted my speech to capture that. Even as Taylor continued to slip, I had a feeling deep in my gut that 2013 would be the year we sprinted forward. This was where two roads diverged. We were racing ahead, and Batten disease was holding my sister back.

I HAD A ten-mile race on the last Saturday in February. It didn't come with the crowds of Thunder Road, and it ended five miles from my parents' house in south Charlotte, so I'd hoped my father could bring Taylor to the finish line. But it was rainy and cold that morning, and my sister had a hard time with extreme temperatures. Dad called when I was lacing up my shoes. "We need to keep T home today," he said. I could hear the disappointment in his voice; my father had come to most of my soccer games, even my rec league games after I graduated from college, and I knew he wanted to watch me finish my race, though not as much as he wanted Taylor to be healthy enough to go outside in bad weather.

"I understand," I said, my voice cracking.

When the gun sounded, I started my watch and glanced down at the old shoes I'd worn because of the rain. They'd been great shoes at one time, but they had more than five hundred miles on them, and the soles were balder than the tires on a junkyard car. I looked at the rain falling out of the sky and figured it wasn't a day for setting personal records.

When the course entered the greenway two miles ahead, my friend Andrew Swistak caught up with me. I'd befriended Andrew, Fletcher's track coach, in recent months even though Taylor no longer went to the school. We'd discovered we lived in the same neighborhood and shared a love for running and clean mountain air. A few days earlier he'd offered to run part of the race with me and pace me to the finish.

"You're making good time," Andrew said, falling into stride beside me. He tapped a few buttons on his watch. "Watch out for the puddle."

I leaped over the standing water covering the boardwalk. "Thanks."

Andrew called out many other puddles on the partially flooded greenway portion of the course. This helped me keep my head up, focus on my form, and hold a steady pace. He talked me through the killer hill at mile eight and coached me on when to pass other runners.

"You know, running is mostly a mind game," he said as we rounded a bend and headed toward the final stretch.

He was right, I knew. Running is all about making adjustments— about knowing how to perform even when elements you can't control, from the weather to your own body, deal you a wild card. Life is like that, too. I started the last climb, and I thought that while I'd taken more than a few hits in the past several years, I was still running. My sister was still running in her own way, too, even if she was too sick to come watch me race in a cold rain—much less chase records. She'd taught me how to keep going on not only the best, but also the worst days.

When I sprinted across the finish line for her, I'd beat all but twenty-six people in the field, and I had my personal record.

I WILL ALWAYS remember the morning we announced our gene therapy grant as if it happened in an alternate universe. Outside the hotel where eighty people had gathered to hear our news, the world was cold and cruel and vast. But inside the banquet hall, I felt warm and safe—euphoric, even. When I stood at the podium and told the crowd about my little sister and the terrible things happening to her, I felt stronger than Batten disease. I heard myself telling them she was blind and couldn't learn like other kids and suffered from seizures. I heard my own words describing how Batten disease would steal her speech and put her in a wheelchair and how I would probably outlive her, even though she was sixteen years younger than me. But up on that podium, none of it felt real. And when I introduced Steve Gray, I believed in the project. I believed in the evolution of gene therapy and the world-class team at UNC and the success of the GAN research. I believed because of Steve's track record and his heart for kids with no hope of a future and, most of all, because of my mother's gut feeling that he was the one.

I could tell our audience believed in Steve, too. He had a way of putting complex science into relatable terms, and the crowd connected with him because of his humble, down-to-earth nature. It was impossible, too, to deny the potential of the work he'd be doing for Batten disease. The enthusiasm in the room was palpable, and immediately following the program people flooded us with hugs and handshakes and promises of support for our mission to save people like Taylor.

"This was amazing," I said to Steve and my father, brother, and John in the parking lot afterward. We were the last ones from the breakfast remaining at the hotel and some of the excitement had started to wane, but I could still feel the smile I'd had all morning in my cheeks.

"It was great," Steve agreed. "I'm excited about getting back to work at the lab." He paused for a moment. "We'll have to be relentless, you know. Nothing worth having is ever easy."

THE MOMENTUM WE'D built in the last days of winter spilled into spring. My body was healthy and strong, and I won awards in almost all of the races I ran. I published several blog posts a week, the words flowing like water. John and I were adding on to our house and planning a dream vacation. Despite the tragedy hanging over our lives like a thundercloud that could burst at any moment, it was a happy time. Meanwhile, my mother rubbed shoulders with representatives of the Michael J. Fox Foundation, the Gates Foundation, and sleek biotech companies at a venture philanthropy conference in April. She and two other Taylor's Tale board members toured the UNC Gene Therapy Center's vector core, the most advanced facility of its kind in the nation. In a nondescript lab down the street from the vector core, Steve and his team kick-started the new gene therapy research for Batten disease.

The first week of May, Mom pulled together the Taylor's Tale board for our annual meeting. Her updates were exciting, but I'd heard most of them already, and when she talked about the funding cycle for the work at UNC, my mind wandered. I watched out the window as the sun dipped behind swollen, purple clouds stacked low on the horizon. My eyes flicked back toward our meeting, and I realized how different the faces around the large conference table looked from the ones who'd sat huddled in a living room with egg salad and pimento cheese sandwiches and copies of *The Cure* the day we first declared war on Batten disease nearly seven years earlier. Yet some of us were still fighting. And now, we were gaining speed.

Two weeks later, my mother flew to Salt Lake City for the annual meeting of the American Society of Gene & Cell Therapy. Her first night away, she called and told me she'd taken Taylor to buy a dress before she left. "She has a dance on Friday," Mom said. "I left the dress hanging on her closet door, and the necklace and earrings are on her dresser. Will you please help your father if he needs it?"

"I can do that," I said, knowing this dance at my sister's new school would be different without her long-time crush, Scott, there to twirl her around the cafeteria floor. It was easier, too, to convince myself this dance would be different because of the new setting instead of Taylor's continued decline, which had made even walking more difficult. But two time zones from home, my mother hadn't forgotten what made my sister happy. I loved her so much in that moment, I wished I could fly to Utah to wrap her in a hug.

ON THE PHONE with me that Friday afternoon, my father was upbeat. "I've got this," he said confidently. "I found your mom's big round brush. Miss T and I are going to turn my bathroom into a beauty shop." I heard Taylor giggle in the background.

"Are you sure?" I asked uncertainly, remembering the "hairstyles" he'd given me on the many nights volunteer work had kept Mom out late during my childhood. I'd envied my brother's short hair then.

"I'm sure," he said. "You and John should go do something fun tonight. I'll send pictures."

"Okay," I said. I didn't tell him that John had already made plans with friends because he thought I'd be busy blow-drying Taylor's hair and applying her tinted lip-gloss, but I didn't want to steal my father's moment. I went to lace up my shoes, deciding it was a perfect night to be outdoors.

Halfway through my run, my cell phone vibrated against my leg. I pulled it out midstride and opened Dad's text with two photos attached. Taylor's thick hair was a little lopsided, but she still looked beautiful in her new sundress and drop earrings, just like I'd known deep down that she would.

My phone safely back in my shorts, I picked up speed, taking deep breaths of air laced with the scent of roses and pine and fresh-cut grass. As I settled into a quick but easy stride, I tried to imagine my sister was running beside me. Instead all I could see was the ugliness of Batten disease. Her latest struggles came rushing at me each time my feet pounded the pavement. I saw her pigeon-toed gait and stiff legs and curled yet rigid hands and wrists. I saw her strained, awkward facial expression, as if she was sucking in her cheeks and slowly rolling her eyes back in her head. I heard her broken speech and the pain in her voice. Batten disease had been whittling away at everything that made my sister whole since the moment she was born, and now it'd broken through.

I used to fight Batten disease like it was a sprint. It took me a long time to learn that Batten disease is more like a marathon. You start off strong, with lots of energy. You have runner's highs and lows. Some days you think you could run forever. But then some days you feel like when you cross the finish line, you'll be so glad to see it—so exhausted—you'll just be happy it's over. Some families, families whose kids have died, had told me in the end it's like that. It's so bad, so freaking ugly, they can't face it anymore. It isn't even about making happy memories at that point. It's about their kid's dignity and their own survival, and about finding peace.

We'd gotten a lot stronger since the beginning. But while I didn't know when the end would be, I'd always be scared of it.

As I ran onto a wide, open street at the far end of my neighborhood, I remembered my sister and Mary-Kate crossing the finish line of the Thunder Road 5K, Taylor clutching the bungee cord, her face turned toward the sky. I was pretty sure it was the most amazing thing I'd ever seen.

And when I started for home, the light just beginning to fade at my back, I knew what I was going to do.

Chapter 20

HELEN KELLER ONCE said that avoiding danger is no safer than exposure. If we always choose the safest path, we aren't truly living. "Security is mostly a superstition," she wrote. "Life is either a daring adventure or nothing."

When I learned about Helen Keller in elementary school, I invented a rudimentary sign language and spelled letters into the palm of my own hand, but the letters never felt the same twice. To experience blindness, I walked the length of the only hallway in our one-story ranch with my eyes squeezed shut until my mother's runner ended beneath my bare feet. I couldn't do the things Helen Keller had done, and that only made her more impressive. I never lost my fascination with her, but I kept my secret language to myself, and I only closed my eyes if I knew it was safe.

I had always imagined blindness would be a horrific thing to endure—one of the reasons I admired my little sister, who'd been nothing but brave. But suddenly, I felt different than I'd ever felt before. I was fearless, fueled by my love for Taylor and my passion for what Taylor's Tale had been trying to do since those early, dark days when my sister could still see light and shadows and sing and dance and run races.

I felt especially fearless when my legs were moving and I could feel the blood pumping in my chest. The idea came to me without warning at the end of my evening run as I realized I wanted, maybe more than anything with the exception of saving Taylor's life, to run a race for her the way *she* had run races—without the gift of sight.

I told John matter-of-factly over dinner that night. "I'm going to run the Thunder Road Half Marathon blindfolded."

"I'm sorry—what?" he said, his fork and knife suspended over his plate.

"I'm running the race blindfolded," I repeated. "For Taylor."

"I heard," John said, spearing a piece of grilled chicken without taking his eyes off me. "How are you going to do that?"

"I'll have a guide," I answered, thinking quickly. I hadn't *thought* much about running blind at all, I realized.

"Who?"

I hesitated. Then, I remembered my pacer for the rain-drenched ten-miler I'd run three months earlier. "Andrew Swistak."

"Has Andrew ever guided a runner wearing a blindfold?"

Silence.

"Have you asked Andrew?"

"I'll talk to him tonight."

"Am I allowed to say I think this is a bad idea?"

"You can say whatever you want," I said, my tone turning stubborn. "I'm running the race blind." But then I realized my husband was doing everything he could not to smile at my persistence.

That night I sent Andrew a message on Facebook. I had a pseudo-crazy idea, and I couldn't pull it off alone. Would he serve as my sighted running buddy to help me mark the five-year anniversary of Taylor's first race?

He answered so quickly, I worried that he didn't understand what I'd asked. Sure, he said—if he was around he'd love to do it, and we should wear purple shirts for Taylor's Tale.

But when Andrew called me a week later, his tone was serious, his words measured. While checking his calendar, he said, he'd started thinking about the prospect of guiding a blind runner for 13.1 miles, even digging up obscure blog posts and articles on the topic. He learned that most runner/guide pairs had been together for years.

"I'll do it on one condition," he said.

"Anything," I answered.

"You have to be okay with falling. Because you *will* fall."

"I'm okay with falling," I repeated, remembering how Taylor had stumbled and scraped her knees during her first race. The threat of a few scrapes and cuts couldn't stop me from doing this now.

"Then I'm in," he said. "Let me know when you want to get started." He paused, and in that moment I wished we'd talked in person, because I was so happy I wanted to hug him. "We should probably begin by walking, just to get used to the tether," Andrew continued. But in my mind, I was already sprinting ahead.

JUNE 5, I BURST into the garage where John was sanding a slab of wood for the bar top in our addition. "I need a tether," I said breathlessly. "Andrew and I are training tonight."

"Okay," my husband said, switching off the sander and setting his safety glasses on the workbench. He turned and rummaged through a drawer for a minute, then held out a short bungee cord, suppressing a grin. "I think you should use this."

"Is that—?"

"It's the one T used in her first race," he said. "I put it away for safekeeping."

I swallowed, the hair standing up on my arms. I took the nondescript, twenty-four-inch length of nylon and draped it over my shoulders. "Thank you," I said, my voice barely a whisper, before I went running down the driveway and into the black night.

I didn't have a blindfold—part of Andrew's plan to start conservatively and focus on getting used to each other. But after a few minutes, he took me to a nearby school's track so we could practice making turns.

"We're protected here," he said, looking around at the fenced-in track and bleachers. "Do you want to give blindness a try?"

A thousand emotions coursed through my body. In the empty stadium I visualized my sister running, determination etched into her face. I saw her being wheeled down the hallway of a faraway hospital en route to an experimental surgery and, more recently, struggling to walk along my parents' street as she clutched the handles of her new walker, sunlight slanting through the trees. Without answering Andrew, I wrapped my fingers tightly around the bungee cord that had been my sister's lifeline and closed my eyes.

The bottom dropped out from under me, reminding me of the feeling I'd get when a roller coaster took its first big dive. My legs turned to Jell-O. I couldn't run in a straight line.

But soon, with Andrew's help, I found my bearings in my dark world. I learned to understand the meaning of my friend's tugs on the tether. I made ninety-degree turns on his spoken direction. It didn't seem possible that any of it was happening, so I didn't try to understand it. After a while, we returned to the neighborhood. I figured out how to change direction and shift to the side for oncoming cars.

I thought I'd mastered running blind—albeit more slowly than I ran sighted—until I mistimed a curb jump and twisted my ankle. Though I kept my balance, the injury served as a painful reminder that *nothing* about blindness is easy, and nothing about our race would be easy.

But nothing about Batten disease or our fight to save people like Taylor came easily, either. And a twisted ankle on my first shot at running blind wasn't going to stop me.

WHILE I HEALED, my mother flew to Washington. Steve Gray's GAN research was going before the Recombinant DNA Advisory Committee. Getting approval from the federal advisory committee was a crucial step toward the first clinical trial for GAN, and the university team and Lori Sames of Hannah's Hope had asked Mom to speak during the public comments section. I watched the live webcast of the hearing on my computer at work.

Mom told the roomful of government scientists about the mission of Taylor's Tale and why we were funding gene therapy research for Batten disease at UNC, though she mostly talked about Taylor. She spoke beautifully, but it was difficult to hear her explain how my sister was losing her independence. She realized she could give up and enjoy the time she had left with her child, she said. But she couldn't stop fighting, because there would always be another Taylor.

I felt a lump forming in my throat as it dawned on me that I'd never heard my mother speak so candidly about my sister's condition. I remembered suddenly that when we'd first started Taylor's Tale, she wouldn't let me use the word "fatal" in any of our communications. "Just say 'life-threatening,'" she told me after I drafted the copy for our first brochure. "Don't say 'fatal.'" But now Batten was ugly and real and we couldn't run away anymore.

"We realize the risk of participating in a trial like this," Mom told the committee in closing. "But we live every day with the knowledge that the consequence of doing nothing for our children is sure and certain death."

As my mother gathered her notes and walked away from the podium, I knew she hadn't been thinking about the Portland stem cell trial or even the GAN trial she was there to support when she wrote her talk. She'd been thinking about the future treatment her own daughter wouldn't live to receive.

The committee granted approval for the GAN work to take the next step toward a gene therapy clinical trial, and I knew Taylor's Tale could help make sure Batten disease wasn't far behind. But right then it was hard to think about what came next in the fight.

I RAN WITH Andrew again the next week, after my ankle had healed; when I closed my eyes, I sprang from the pavement and into the blackness, with all of the shakiness from that first night gone. When we practiced again two days later, we were faster. I kept my eyes squeezed shut, but I could see the flashing red of the caution light in the center of our neighborhood when we ran beneath it. I guessed our direction, because I could feel the grade of the road and knew it sloped downward away from the clubhouse.

"I need a blindfold," I said to Andrew without breaking stride. "Taylor can't see that light." The next time we ran, I used a bandana to make a makeshift blindfold. The fabric was thin, and on subsequent runs I found that I still had to close my eyes to block out all of the light, but I was closer to seeing the world the way my little sister saw it.

WHILE I BECAME a blind runner, my mother tended to our charity's needs and adjusted to Taylor's increasing care needs. She kept up with Steve Gray and worked the international advocacy circuit from her tablet and smartphone as she measured Taylor's medications and took her to pool therapy and managed part-time caregivers. Once upon a time Mom and I had taken frequent walks, but now Taylor's Tale and my sister's medical needs kept her so busy she didn't have time for herself. That's why she surprised me when she shared her plan for Thunder Road.

"I can't do a half marathon blindfolded, but I'm going to run the 5K," she announced suddenly while we were washing dishes after dinner at my parents' house one night. "For T."

"That's great," I said, but silently I worried about my mother, who was slender but had never been athletic and was closer to sixty than fifty. "I'll coach you," I added after a moment. "If you want."

"I'd like that." She smiled, laugh lines lighting up the soft blush on her cheeks.

"You'll be terrific," I said, and I meant it. "Plus, it'll mean a lot to have you there on race day."

"What's it like?" she asked.

"Running?" I smiled. "It's not so bad."

ANDREW HAD PROMISED I'd fall, and I did, on a sticky night in August three days before Taylor's fifteenth birthday. We'd scarcely made it up the hill from my cul-de-sac when my shoe caught the curb. I could almost hear my ligaments and bones crunching and grinding as my ankle went left and right and left again. My body tumbled into a black void as I lost my balance. I didn't have time to rip off my blindfold, so instinct took over. I threw out my right hand to catch my fall, and seconds later Andrew was helping me up from my sprawled position on the side of the street. I was still wearing the blindfold, but I felt warm blood oozing from my left knee, and my right palm burned where I'd scraped it on the pavement. I tied the blindfold around my leg to keep the blood from trickling onto my shoe before limping back to the house.

"I guess we'll call it a night," Andrew said, holding the door for me as I untied my shoes.

"I'm not done," I answered, brushing asphalt out of the wound on my knee. "Give me a few minutes to clean up, and we'll head back out."

We ran the equivalent of a 5K after my spill, and I couldn't help but think that Taylor would have done the same thing.

I RAN A sighted 5K for my sister on her birthday and wrote a blog post about it, leaving just enough time before the party to shower and load up the back of my car with gifts.

Stephen was in the parking lot when John and I arrived at my family's favorite Italian restaurant. John nodded at him and walked inside to get a table.

"How's the blind running going?" Stephen asked, giving me a hug.

"It's unlike anything else," I answered. "A few weeks ago we ran in the rain. I'd never really *felt* raindrops on my skin like that before. Blindness changes everything."

"I'm glad I can see," my brother said softly.

I blinked in the bright August sun and tried to focus on my younger brother. He was tall and solid, and his dark hair had blond streaks from hours of riding bikes on high mountain trails. He had a good job and a steady girlfriend and plenty of friends. I thought about how much had fallen into place for me, too. I'd stumbled across a new career opportunity that summer and expected to get an offer any day. I had solid friendships and a loving family and a nice roof over my head. I'd vacationed in some of the most beautiful places on Earth, all before I turned thirty. Outside of Batten disease, life was good.

But it could just as easily have been us. I'd had carrier testing six months after the diagnosis; Stephen had waited six years, but we'd received the same result. I'll never forget the somber tone in my doctor's voice the day she called with my report, as if somebody had died. "Don't feel sorry for me," I'd said, thinking of the ticking time bomb in my sister's body. "I didn't get Batten disease."

"Do you ever wonder what it would be like? If it had been you?"

Stephen looked at the ground. "Sometimes."

"I think about it all the time; I think about how I got one good copy and one bad copy of the Batten disease gene, and she got two bad copies." I paused. "After everything, it's still hard for me to swallow that a single roll of the dice is the difference between living and dying."

He was silent for a moment. Then, finally, "I can't believe T's fifteen."

Now, I blinked back tears. "I wish time would slow down. Every time she celebrates a birthday, she's sicker."

I sat next to the guest of honor. Taylor didn't join our conversation, though she laughed at Stephen and John's jokes. As we all talked around her at her own birthday party, I thought about how I hadn't spoken *with* my sister in a long time, because Batten disease was stealing her speech. I realized I didn't know how she felt, what she wanted, or what she would say if we could chat the way most sisters do. I thought that while Batten disease hadn't taken my sister's life yet, Batten disease had already stolen my sister.

Later at my parents' house for dessert, I got choked up reading birthday cards from Taylor's friends at Fletcher, who hadn't forgotten her more than a year after her departure from the school; a boy named Paul and his mom had delivered the cards and pink-frosted cupcakes that afternoon. As the hour grew late, Mom carried out the cake, and Dad lit the candles. My mother wrapped an arm around Taylor; as we sang the notes to "Happy Birthday," I noticed Mom had an odd catch in her voice.

ANDREW'S SECOND SON was born in the dog days of summer, and baby duty made it difficult for us to plan training runs. Though we'd fared well on near-empty neighborhood streets after dark, I knew a half marathon course with other runners would be different. I needed more practice.

"I'll run with you," John said matter-of-factly one night while we were watching TV—rare downtime.

"You will?" I raised my eyebrows. My husband had once told me he'd rather dig a ditch than go for a run.

"Sure. If Andrew's busy I'll stand in for a couple of turns."

"It's not easy," I said.

"Nothing worth having is easy—right?" He grinned. "Come on. We'll take it slow."

John and I made it through our first tethered run that night without any falls—and then our second, and our third. We didn't have a handle on spacing or bungee cord tension or timing for turns the way Andrew and I did, but we survived. And because our lack of experience forced us to slow down, I "saw" more of the world. A divot in the pavement. The sound of voices in backyards. Autumn whispering in the leaves of trees after the last of the late-summer heat died with the setting sun.

IT'D BEEN ALMOST two years since my ambulance ride and brief hospital stay for a frightening migraine, but John hadn't forgotten my vow to take better care of myself. In September he whisked me away to Wyoming for ten days of hiking in the Grand Tetons and Yellowstone. I'd accepted the job with a marketing agency and resigned from the hospital after eight years, just a few days before we left. I hoped the change would mean more focused work and less stress at the office. Excited for a fresh start, I felt energized and carefree as we boarded the plane. Later that day I said a prayer to God as I laced up my ankle braces and top-of-the-line boots, dug my poles into the dirt, and hiked my first miles on my balky joints. The race of my life was eight weeks away.

We hiked sixty miles on the trip. Some were relaxing, while some tested my endurance, my wasted ankles, and the muscles in my legs. But the rewards—the wildlife and the sweeping views and the clean mountain air—made every tough mile worth the effort. All that beauty gave me strength for the endless switchbacks. I hoped our fight against Batten disease would be like that, in the end. Some days Batten knocked us down and kicked dirt in our faces and rubbed rocks in our wounds. But hearing my sister laugh on her birthday and feeling the warmth in her hand and believing we could make a difference for future Taylors made all that pain more bearable somehow.

I called my parents one night while I was icing my ankles on the porch of our cabin in Jackson. My mother put Taylor on the phone. I told her about the bull moose we'd seen in the woods, describing his chocolate skin and huge rack of antlers and how lazy he'd been, just sitting around chewing on grass in the trees while people took pictures of him. My sister couldn't respond, but Mom told me that was the first time Taylor laughed all day.

After I said goodbye, I thought that while I'd had fun describing the moose to my sister, I wished she could have seen it for herself. While I took the trip of a lifetime, Taylor sat on our parents' sofa, waiting for her big sister to call and tell her about sights and sounds and experiences she could only dream about.

When I went to sleep that night, I was ready to go home and keep fighting.

AUTUMN SEEMED TO pass as quickly as dry leaves in a gust of wind. Andrew and I began training together again. The Taylor's Tale board and community of supporters had rallied around the run; nearly sixty people had registered to run the half marathon or 5K for our team, ranging from family and close friends to members of a teen service organization called Playing for Others. Taylor was part of the organization's buddy program, and the kids, many of them her age, had grown to love her that fall.

Meanwhile, the media's interest in our effort caught fire. The daily and weekly newspapers and the local television stations ran stories. We were featured on popular running blogs and landed the cover story of *Endurance Magazine,* a statewide fitness publication. I did phone interviews on my morning commute, and Andrew and I ran short circuits in parking lots and city parks for news cameras on our lunch break. Nine days before the race of my life, a freelancer with *Runner's World* contacted me for an interview. Though I'd pitched the story to the magazine's editor weeks earlier, I didn't believe the email was real. I only responded to the writer after I Googled her name.

ANDREW AND I chose a quiet Saturday morning for our last practice session. Running in darkness as the morning fog lifted to reveal a bright, sunny day, I felt the sensation of cars as they passed us on the road, even though they moved to the center lane to give us space. I felt the corrugated texture of a bridge when we crossed the interstate and the painted white lines on the road, still slick with dew.

At some point, Andrew asked if I wanted to run untethered.

"What?" I asked cautiously, remembering the accident that had left my knee bloodied in August. I quickly tried to count the cars I'd heard on our run that morning. "Here?"

"We're on a side road without any traffic right now," he said. "This is your chance."

There was no turning back. My legs and my heart wanted and needed to do this, I realized. And without a word, I nodded, taking hold of both ends of the bungee cord that had been my lifeline for five months and my sister's five years earlier. I located the white stripes painted down the center of the street with the soles of my shoes. I settled into my stride and picked up my speed, and I felt free as a bird. I found myself silently talking to God. I asked Him to take care of my sister, because that's what He'd done for me.

I was running untethered, but never alone. And I didn't fall.

I was ready.

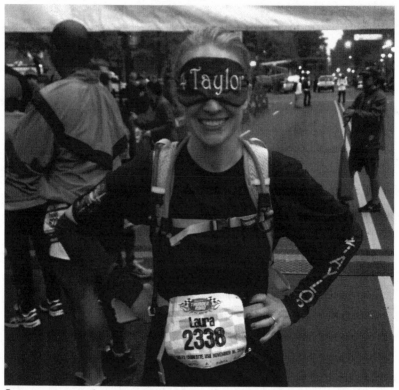

Laura arrives at the starting line of the race of her life, 2013

Chapter 21

THE MORNING OF a race is like nothing else. The exhilaration of hearing the gun and crossing the timing mats and darting ahead of other bodies, their legs and arms churning to keep up, can't be replicated on a training run.

But as I laced my shoes and wrote my sister's name on my arm and draped the bungee cord around my shoulders in the stillness of my house, I felt an unbelievable sense of peace. It was as if I'd paddled beyond the waves crashing on the shore, and now I was floating in the calm. I could see crowds on the beach and sharks in the shallows, but out here I was alone—and I wasn't afraid.

It was still dark when we arrived uptown, and streetlamps cast pools of light on the pavement. Other runners were just beginning to trickle into the city center from parking lots and decks and light rail stations. They drifted down sidewalks in running shirts and visors like clusters of multicolored ghosts.

A TV news crew and a magazine photographer were waiting for me at the start line. They asked if I was nervous and if I thought I'd run a fast race and if my sister would be able to come to the finish line. I smiled and answered their questions without really hearing them, like someone else was in my body. Most of my family and one hundred of my closest friends would be at the race. But Batten disease was strong and my sister was too sick to come. In an hour a caregiver would arrive at my parents' house to stay with Taylor so my father could join us uptown. I told the reporters my sister was brave. I didn't tell them Batten disease was winning the war for my sister.

A few minutes after sunrise, I hugged my mother and John goodbye and walked to the starting line with Andrew and Steve Gray, who'd driven to Charlotte from Chapel Hill the previous night. Steve ran races when he wasn't studying devastating diseases in his lab or raising his three children, and weeks earlier he'd asked if he could run Thunder Road with us. I couldn't think of a better runner to share the road with my guide and me than the scientist I believed would discover an answer for people battling Batten disease.

We were starting with the walkers thirty minutes ahead of a stampede of thousands of runners. The early start time option was a new feature and a blessing for us; despite our success in training, Andrew had been firm that starting in the crowd was too dangerous.

I took one end of the bungee cord, feeling the rough nylon and the curved metal hook in the palm of my hand. I pulled down the new blindfold bearing my sister's name. The gun sounded. I ran into darkness.

We quickly left the walkers behind. A policeman charged with pacing the early starters drove a truck at the head of the field. We tried to pass him, and I heard him yelling at Andrew. But the words they exchanged were watery, drowned out by the rhythmic sound of my soles hitting the street. The policeman was slowing us down, but it didn't matter. My legs were begging to sprint, but for the first time since I'd started running races, my mind wasn't focused on my speed. Taylor had never cared about being fast. She had only cared about crossing the finish line.

I hadn't set out to run for speed, but suddenly the situation with the pace car frustrated me. We were almost walking now. We'd trained for months and worked hard to rally support, and now one person stood in our way.

"Let's just go," I said. Things don't always happen as planned, I thought as I quickened my pace. I expected to have a healthy sister. I expected to have a smooth race. People said Taylor couldn't run blind. They said we couldn't beat Batten disease. Now this officer said we couldn't run our race. He was just another voice I'd choose to ignore.

"We took a wrong turn," Andrew told us after we left the pace car behind and shot ahead of the course markers. I didn't respond, instead turning and running with my guide in the opposite direction when he tugged on the bungee cord.

Someone shouted my name from far away. Then I heard my name again, closer this time, as if the owner of the voice had sprinted to catch up with us. I kept running. I felt the November sun on my face as it climbed in the sky. The road widened after we left the pace car behind. We picked up speed.

I found my stride on the open, near-deserted course, and for the first time I thought about the whirlwind days leading up to the race. I'd delivered purple shirts to runners and walkers on our team and banners to our cheer station captains. My new coworkers had given me a surprise pep rally on Friday; they'd worn purple for Taylor and lured me to the lobby with a fake delivery, then blasted the *Rocky* theme song and taken pictures and made a donation to Taylor's Tale. At the race expo that afternoon, I'd discovered all of the pre-race media had turned me into a minor celebrity among other runners.

Now, the world was dark and it was just Andrew and Steve and I and an invisible race course stretching out for miles ahead of us.

Something strange happened then. After we broke away from the police officer in the truck, we maintained a near-record pace for me despite the blindfold. I could feel my heart beating in my chest and the muscles working in my legs, and running was more effortless than it had ever been. I soared over speed bumps and manhole covers and zigzagged through winding neighborhood roads. Later I learned from race photos that I'd even split photographers perched on tall stepladders.

We'd left the walkers far behind, and we were alone on the course for a long time before the race leaders caught up with us. I couldn't see, but my ears told a story. Each time we approached a cheer station, set up at approximately one-mile intervals along the course, people voiced encouragement as they would for any runner. Then, they went silent as they realized I was blindfolded. "I wish you could see the looks on their faces," Andrew said as we approached one station. But I didn't need to see them. I could hear them clapping and jumping up and down and yelling encouragement long after we'd run past them.

It was my race. It was Taylor's race. And nothing had ever felt so wonderful in my life.

WHEN ANDREW SAID we were entering a tree-lined street of stately homes, I knew we weren't far from the finish line. A few miles ahead, a throng of friends stood at the race's final turn, waiting for us. But I didn't want it to end.

For months I had told people I wanted my sister to be the first person I saw when I took off my blindfold. But as summer became autumn and I transformed into a blind runner, it'd become clear that navigating the crowded city streets on race day would be too difficult for Taylor. In the five months since I'd first run in the dark, my sister had slipped farther down into the dark chasm of Batten disease. I was strong and healthy and had adjusted quickly to "losing" my vision, but Batten disease had stolen my sister's legs; by that fall she struggled to walk, even with a walker. It was stealing her voice, too. Reporters had asked me how my sister felt about my attempt to run a half marathon blindfolded. I always hated saying, "I wish she could tell me." She suffered from myoclonic seizures, like a thousand little electric jolts that made her body twitch and jerk.

Andrew spoke then. "Do you want to run untethered again?" His voice sounded far away. I nodded. Andrew and Steve dropped behind me, and I was alone in the tunnel of trees. My gait felt smooth, my body weightless, my breathing effortless. I thought maybe I could run forever. I touched the only photo that existed of Taylor finishing her first race, attached to my armband. It felt both heavy and light on my arm.

In my mind I saw my sister, swinging beneath the grand old oaks in our parents' backyard. I saw her short honey hair and baby teeth in perfect rows and eyes the color of caramel, twinkling in the soft afternoon light. *Higher*, she said, *higher!* She pumped her tiny legs and the swing swung higher and higher until her feet almost touched heaven.

It felt like a dream.

But it wasn't.

WE APPROACHED THE cheer station at the final turn. We ran under the bridge where I'd seen the blind runner three years earlier. I gave Andrew the bungee cord one more time. Untethered, I quickened my pace. I heard the screams and shouts and cowbells of one hundred friends and relatives and the Playing for Others teenagers. The sounds melted the cramps in my legs and filled my heart with love. In front of the crowd, I made a ninety-degree turn on Andrew's spoken direction alone. We headed for the end.

Andrew kept the tether as we approached the finish line. The world was silent again. I never heard the seventy teens from our cheer station sprinting down the finish chute beside us, chanting my name.

I hurdled over the first raised timing mat, and then the second, and Andrew pulled me to a stop before my momentum sent me crashing into a line of people I couldn't see. As I lifted my blindfold and let the light come pouring in, I melted into the arms of my mother, who'd been waiting for me. She was crying, and I realized I was crying, too. The crowd surrounded us then, closing us off from the outside world.

Even though I had a medal around my neck and a timing chip on my shoe, I wasn't at a race any longer, and I didn't care that I'd just run a half marathon blindfolded. In that moment, I didn't hate Batten disease, because I wasn't thinking about Batten disease at all. Emotion and love washed over me and I understood the gift I'd received.

We stayed there for a long time, clogging the finish chute, protected by a ring of kids in purple tutus and pompoms and t-shirts holding homemade signs. We were breaking the rules, but none of the race officials seemed to care.

Five years ago Taylor had crossed the finish line here. But five years is a long time. And well before she became a runner, my sister was already dying.

When the writer with *Runner's World* interviewed me, she asked if I thought running a half marathon blindfolded could save my sister. But I'd been fighting for future Taylors for years.

I'D RUN 13.1 miles in the dark. But I didn't take a single step alone.

As I ran the final stretch of Thunder Road, led by the voice of a friend and the courage of a dying girl, I understood: Batten disease may have cast a dark shadow on our world, but I wasn't running away any longer.

I was running to the light.

I believed.

And I felt free.

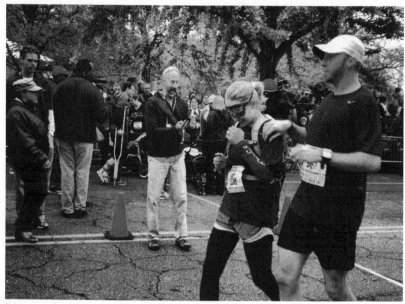

Laura and Andrew cross the finish line, 2013

Epilogue

I wanted to write this epilogue long before I'd finished the final chapter of *Run to the Light*. Now, however, I realize I don't know how to talk about my sister in an essay most people won't read until at least ten months from now. What will life look like then? Should I refer to Taylor in the present tense, or past?

Here's the thing: my sister is dying and I've had eleven years to get used to the idea and I'm still not comfortable with it, and I can't help her and I don't know what to do. Sometimes, when I'm having a rough day, I think that after Taylor is gone, I'll want to pick up my life and move somewhere far away from home.

But I know better than to believe that I can run away from my own agony. I've tried that trick, and it doesn't work. Real pain doesn't dwell in a single physical location. It exists in the heart and the mind and the soul. It'd be easier to let it all wash away, gone forever, like sandcastles at the changing of the tide. But if that ever happened, a large part of me would be gone forever, too.

If you want to vanquish fear, you have to run toward it.

In one respect, *Run to the Light* had a fairytale ending. What began as a single spark—some might even say a crazy lark of an idea—produced a dreamlike day that fueled a movement and, in its own way, saved my life. I remember the Thunder Road race as if it happened only moments ago. Though I haven't run blind in a long time, I can still feel the cold metal hook of the bungee cord in my clenched hand and the subtle dips and rises of the earth beneath my feet and my mother's hot tears on my cheek at the finish line. Born out of a tragedy, it was an incredible experience I'll never forget.

But Taylor was already struggling then. And a few years after I crossed the finish line at Thunder Road, Taylor was admitted to the hospital when her seizures spiraled out of control. The doctors intubated her. The hospital staff called hospice and palliative care. Mom and Dad suffered on their own separate islands, one resigned to making her comfortable, the other determined to keep her alive. I watched and waited and kept my own feelings locked inside.

Taylor, of course, shocked everyone and went home after twelve days. Though she returned to the hospital several times over the course of that year, she didn't go back after starting the ketogenic diet—a high-fat, adequate-protein, low-carbohydrate meal plan that forces the body to burn fats and can massively reduce seizure activity.

Meanwhile, the little engine of Taylor's Tale kept going. In the years since Thunder Road, Taylor's Law established the nation's first rare disease advisory council in North Carolina. A clinical-stage biopharmaceutical company called Abeona Therapeutics acquired Steve Gray's work on infantile Batten disease. The treatment we believed in and fought for is becoming a reality, and the first clinical trial could begin before this book is published.

As for myself, I still try to live my life by the lessons I learned in the dark that day at Thunder Road. Running blind taught me to view any bad situation as a noble challenge, rather than an impassable wall. It taught me to see that overcoming obstacles, however big or small, can be achieved by changing our perspective. By believing we can turn tragedy into opportunity. Believing that while today may make us cry or scream, tomorrow is our second chance. I survived because I learned to see the world like Taylor.

After I took off the blindfold, I realized I wasn't done running for my sister: now I'm completing a race in all fifty states. And in 2017, I achieved something I'd never believed I was capable of doing: I gave a TED talk—essentially a fifteen-minute version of this book—in front of a packed house.

As I write this, Taylor is stable—for her. While the ketogenic diet proved to be magical for seizure control, her quality of life is almost nonexistent. On a good day, Mom can make her laugh by singing a silly song. Those laughs, and her muted cries of pain or discomfort, are the only signs that my sister is still here, a prisoner in her own broken body. Observing Taylor's special brand of existence the past several years has made me question my own definition of quality. What is it? Who gets to determine it? When is a person's life still worth living? When is it not?

I don't know the answers, and maybe that's why, these days, I measure life not in years or days, but in the lives we change. My sister's life here on Earth, whenever it ends, has been spent far differently than anything most of us will ever know. But her life has been one of love, strength, dedication, and hope. It will be far too short, but the world won't soon forget its impact. And one day, after we're both long gone, her courage will live on, in the pages of this book, the law that bears her name, the potential treatment for future Taylors, and the hearts and minds and souls of the many, many people she's touched.

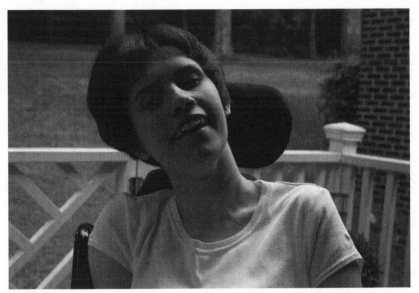

Taylor, 2017

Acknowledgements

Thank you:

To Carin Siegfried, who urged me to write this book and gave me the courage to share my story with more raw emotion and less control.

To Betsy Thorpe and Karen Alley, whose suggestions made the manuscript better.

To draft readers Jen Band, Jesica D'Avanza, John Edwards, Judy Goldman, Bo Hussey, Ricki Lewis, Amy Marsh, Ruth Moose, Marlee Murphy, Linda Phillips, Leah Shearer, Jen Stephens, Shannon Swiger, Bart Yasso, and Alex Zsoldos.

To Steve Gray, David Jones, and Ricki Lewis, for making sure I didn't mess up the science.

To Claudia Wilde and C.A. Casey, for believing in *Run to the Light*, and to everyone on the Bink Books team, for sharing it with the world.

To Bill Baker, Laura Tice, and Rusty Williams, for your artistic talents and time.

To my longtime piano teacher, Dzidra Reimanis, for buying my first short story for a dollar the year I turned five.

To my fourth grade teacher, Miss Wilson, for celebrating my weirdness when I wanted to scribble words in spiral notebooks during recess, while everyone else played four square and red light, green light.

To Mrs. Blackburn, my ninth grade English teacher, for giving me the C that made me work harder.

To Susan Ketchin, for making me feel like a real writer when I was broken and scared.

To the Taylor's Tale volunteers and friends who stood by us in our refusal to take "no cure" for an answer.

To John Crowley, for showing us how it's done.

To children and families everywhere fighting Batten disease.

To the scientists and clinicians who work around the clock to make life better and longer for current and future patients.

To the faculty, staff, and students of The Fletcher School, for providing a safe, loving space for Taylor to grow for six years.

To Charlotte Frank, Callie Lloyd, Nicole McEwen, and Scott Wallace, for being true friends to my sister.

To Mary-Kate Behnke and Andrew Swistak, for guiding a blind runner to the finish line.

To the TEDxCharlotte team, for giving me fifteen minutes on that stage.

To my family, for supporting me.

To Daisy, for making sure my office never feels too lonely.

To my Grandma Kathryn, for teaching me that adversity makes you strong.

To my mother, for inspiring me.

To my husband, John, for filling in fifteen years of memories to help me write this book, and for loving me.

To Taylor, for being.